# A PATIENT-CENTERED APPROACH FOR THE CHRONICALLY-ILL

Irene S. Switankowsky

University Press of America,® Inc.
Lanham · Boulder · New York · Toronto · Plymouth, UK

**Copyright © 2016 by**
**University Press of America,® Inc.**
4501 Forbes Boulevard
Suite 200
Lanham, Maryland 20706
UPA Acquisitions Department (301) 459-3366

Unit A, Whitacre Mews, 26-34 Stannary Street,
London SE11 4AB, United Kingdom

Library of Congress Control Number: 2015943496
ISBN: 978-0-7618-6626-8 (paperback : alk. paper)
eISBN: 978-0-7618-6627-5

# Contents

## Part I

## Part II

# Part I

# Chapter 1

# Introduction

The patient-centered approach that I advocate in this book is especially suited to the chronically-ill. The chronically-ill patient is anything but your *typical* patient. This type of patient needs a lot of *guidance and advice* on how to self-manage his/her life. And there are no guarantees for the patient to manage her symptoms either. So, providing medical care for these kinds of patients can be very difficult and time consuming. But it is the only way physicians can most effectively treat chronic illness.

This book is divided into two main parts. In Part I, I describe the type of patient-care that is required for most chronically-ill patients. In this section, I argue that the chronically-ill patient is very different from an acutely-ill patient who simply has a problem which can be alleviated by surgery or medication. The nature of chronic illness usually continues for a patient's lifetime. So, there are no conclusive medications or straight forward treatments that will alleviate the patient's symptoms once and for all. It can be very hard for the physician to treat such patients, given the increasing time constraints that are inherent in medical practice on all levels.

Therefore, I will argue that there are things that patients can do for themselves to make the clinical encounter easier. It is not merely up the physician to do all the hard work for the patient. Despite the constant pain and fatigue that the chronically-ill patient feels, (s)he must still take consistent steps to manage his/her health (with the help of the physician). In other words, the patient still has to take care of him/herself and make his/her life the best that it could be, given his/her physical disabilities.

There are also psychological ramifications of chronic illness which have to be dealt with directly by the patient and other medical specialists. The patient may want to seek alternative therapies as well, such as psychologists, massage therapists, acupuncturists, and physiotherapists. But in addition to all of these medical and alternative measures, the patient him/herself must also become proactive in dealing with the illness and take steps to make sure that (s)he lives the best possible life.

In Chapter 3, I discuss the patient-related problems of dealing with a chronic illness. Patients have responsibilities for taking care of their chronic illness as well to the physician. Self-management is crucially important for any chronically-ill patient. It is not merely the physician who has responsibilities to the patient. The patient has to comply with treatments, accept his/her illness, take medications as prescribed, gain control over his/her symptoms by problem-solving, and being an active self-manager. This will help the physician best treat the patient.

In Chapter 4, I discuss the physician-related problems with treating a chronic illness. Most chronic illnesses are not measurable and cannot be assessed in these ways. Therefore, physicians must cope with the unpredictable nature of chronic illness and the ways in which different patients cope with the illness. Each patient will cope with the chronic illness very differently. This can substantially complicate the clinical encounter and makes it extremely unpredictable. I argue that by following the four conditions outlined in Part II the physician can advocate patient-centered medicine, the type of medicine that is most relevant and successful for the chronically-ill patient.

Therefore, Chapter 5 focuses on the first condition of the patient-centered approach which focuses on how to bring about empathic communication. It is very important for the physician to communicate clearly and empathically with the chronically-ill patient. This can really help the physician to most effectively understand the patient's predicament and help the physician come to terms with the symptoms of a chronic illness.

In Chapter 6, I focus on the second condition which is effective physician-patient understanding. One important aspect of this condition is to ensure that the physician has a proper understanding of the patient's unique difficulties and disabilities. This can take a lot of probing over time, but it is the only way to most effectively bring about the patient-centered approach one in which the physician can best comprehend a patient's predicament and how (s)he can best help the patient.

In Chapter 7, I focus on the third condition of the patient-centered approach which is successful decision-making. Chronically-ill patients can become very negative and may start framing all of their experiences of illness in black and white terms. This condition requires that the physician rationally *guide* the patient's medical decisions so that they are reasonable. The last thing a physician needs is to realize that the patient made an irrational decision in favor or against treatment. This is why a certain amount of monitoring by the physician is necessary.

In Chapter 8, I focus on the fourth condition of the patient-centered approach which focuses on the development of a trusting physician-patient relationship. Trust is a very important part of patient care and which requires empathy. It can take a long time to develop a relationship of mutual trust and respect between physician and patient. But it is necessary to develop an open-honest physician-patient relationship so that patient-centered care can be effectively administered.

The four conditions of the patient-centered approach outlined above underlie the most humane approach to medical care for the chronically-ill and make it possible for the physician to care for such patients in the best possible way. I discuss the parameters of the humane patient-centered approach in Chapter 9 and why it is important to advocating an effective physician-patient approach that makes the patient central to the medical interaction.

Lastly, in the Chapter 10, I discuss the unpredictable nature of chronic illness. It is very important for the physician and patient to realize that there are no cures to chronic illness and that life is an uphill battle for a chronically ill patient, except when the illness stabilizes and the patient doesn't become more disabled for a while. So, it is important for both the patient and physician to understand and accept this unpredictability as part of treating and dealing with a chronic condition.

In the Appendix, I offer a tool for patients to use manage chronic illness by becoming an effective self-manager. I believe that it is in self-management that the patient can help to reduce time for the physician. The patient will have to live with this disease for the rest of his/her life. So, it is of upmost importance for the individual to learn as many techniques as possible to help him/herself live the best possible life with arthritis, or any other chronic condition.

At this point, I would like to include a caveat. In this book, most times I discuss arthritis as a chronic illness. This is because I have most experience and information with the disease having it myself and also leading many arthritis workshops for over a decade in all areas of South-western Ontario. But the same types of self-management skills can be applied to all chronic illnesses and very similar issues arise for medical practitioners and patients.

Chronic illness can be very hard to cope with for the patient. But it is also hard for the physician to treat such a long-term illness because of the time that it takes to effectively help the patient. The medical care required for chronic illness is individual and completely patient-specific. In addition, each patient will be able to proactively cope with his/her illness in varying degrees. Because of these idiosyncrasies, it is important for the physician and patient to each do his/her part in treating the illness.

My hope is that this book will help both the physician to most effectively treat a chronic illness and the patient to better manage chronic the symptoms and disabilities of the illness. There are no easy answers, and there are many ambiguities and complexities. But it is possible for a chronically-ill patient to live a good life, one that is not filled with so much pain and disability by managing his/her life. Then the physician can help *guide* the patient to live that best life. This is ideally the purpose of the patient-centered approach for the chronically-ill patient advocated in this book.

# Chapter 2

# The Nature of Chronic Illness

## Introduction

Chronic illness usually consists of a complicated web of symptoms. Some of these symptoms are related to fatigue, often because the patient is overwhelmed by a lack of sleep. Other times, the symptoms involve a sense of loss of control because of constant pain and disability. Since many of a chronic patient's symptoms involve the psychophysical aspects of the disease itself, they cannot be alleviated by the physician in any straightforward manner. Psychophysical symptoms involve the physical *and* psychological aspects of illness. In chronic illness, the consistency of the physical symptoms and disabilities can lead to depression and a lack of well-being because of the continuation of pain and the increasing disabilities of chronically-ill patients. They are simply conditions that the patient must deal with consistently because of the nature of chronic illness. All patients can hope for is that the symptoms be controlled to some degree and they could have a better quality of life from time to time.

Given the nature of chronic illness, it may even be difficult for a patient to clearly describe his/her symptoms. The physician may have to do a lot of detective work to determine how the patient can best be helped. There are no easy answers or magical cures for chronic illness. All the physician can do is to offer some relief from the patient's physical symptoms so that (s)he can could enjoy a better quality of life by developing a realistic lifestyle through self-management. I will discuss self-management in more detail in Part II and in the Appendix of the book. Thus, much of what needs to be done to relieve the patient's physical symptoms has to be done by the patient. The physician's role is, therefore, to offer advice and encouragement. The unreliable nature of the physician–patient relationship for chronic illness is very different from the predictable nature of acute illness in medical practice.

Several aspects of chronic illness make it especially difficult for an effective interaction between physician and patient. I will examine these aspects below. Typically, for acute illness, the nature of medical practice is such that physicians usually treat patients for acute symptoms by coming to some sort of resolution and cure for a patient's illness. That is the way acute illnesses are usually dealt with. However, resolution-based treatments are not an effective method for treating chronic illness because this type of illness has no one resolution and is plagued with ambiguity and uncertainty. In addition, the nature of chronic illness is such that no one treatment fits all patients with similar symptoms. This underscores the frustrating nature of chronic illness, both for the patient and physician.

## Acute Medical Practice

Given the nature of normal, acute medical practice, there are several reasons physicians don't feel comfortable telling patients that there is very little that they can do to help them. First, medical practice prides itself on being able to resolve a patient's medical problems since medicine is, at least in part, a science through which certain physical symptoms of the illness are relieved. However, to treat chronically-ill patients, it is essential for physicians to shift this focus from *curing* patients to simply *caring* for them.

Second, the nature of chronic illness is unpredictable since a patient's pain and fatigue usually don't go away. Physicians may sometimes feel as if they're hitting their head against an impenetrable wall of elusive symptoms. In some cases, it's even difficult for a physician to clearly determine the nature of the patient's symptoms. This is because some chronically-ill patients may have a difficult time describing their symptoms in measurable terms. This is because sometimes, words cannot accurately capture the type of pain a patient feels, much less its intensity. This can further hinder effective communication and fragment the physician–patient encounter.

Third, physicians have to deal with a patient's chronic illness for many years. The longevity of the care required can make physicians feel quite overwhelmed. This is to be expected because of the nature of the care that chronically-ill patients require. This type of illness encourages the patient and physician to develop a relationship of understanding, mutual trust, and respect that can last for many years.

## Chronic Medical Practice

How a patient deals with his/her chronic illness depends on several conditions. First, the severity of the disabilities caused by the illness can make a substantial difference on how the patient copes. For instance, if a patient cannot walk without pain, (s)he will have an especially hard time coping with the illness and may even feel hopeless.

Second, a patient who is in constant pain will put all his/her time and energy into finding relief from everyday symptoms. This can negatively impact a person's outlook as well as quality of life. So, the patient may not have any extra energy to effectively cope with some of the other dimensions of the illness, such as the psychological impacts of the illness and some of the prolonged secondary physical and psychological effects of the illness.

Third, some chronically-ill patients feel socially isolated because of their pain and the lack of support that they face in their family. This is to be expected at first because chronic illness does not have physical and observable aspects that family members could see. Most of the symptoms that a chronically-ill patient feels are hidden for the most part. So, at first, family members may be a bit suspicious of a patient telling them that they are too sore or fatigued to do something with the family yet again. Thus, patients may need to develop different types of social support networks to help them overcome their isolation. Isolation is the prime cause of depression and hopelessness among the chronically-ill and these can exacerbate a patient's symptoms and overall outlook.

Lastly, the patient's pre-illness personality can greatly affect the quality of life and how (s)he will deal with his/her pain, fatigue and disability. For instance, if the patient has always been hopeful and upbeat before becoming chronically-ill, (s)he will probably find positive ways to cope with the illness. However, if the patient is naturally hopeless and negative before becoming chronically-ill, (s)he won't have the patience to effectively cope with the onset of the chronic illness and may become increasingly bitter and even depressed.

The nature of chronic illness is such that the patient will probably lose immediate physical strength and be deprived of a pain-free future. In addition, a patient's future is usually marked by continual weakness and disability, which can cause the patient a lot of psychological uncertainty. This unpredictability can make it difficult for a chronically-ill patient to deal with the day-to-day concerns related to the disease over the long-term. There seems to be no reprieve from the malaise of continuous pain and fatigue. Every day becomes an increasingly complex winding road leading to nowhere better.

As a result, even the most upbeat chronically-ill patients can start feeling hopeless and helpless after a while. Many chronically-ill patients feel that they can't do as much as they used to. This hopelessness can make the patient feel even more isolated and depressed. But central to any type of wellness program is learning how to adapt to the illness. Instead of feeling helpless and hopeless all the time, the chronically-ill patient should strive to become more flexible, and develop a positive attitude in relation to his/her disabilities.

It is crucially important for a chronically-ill patient to create and sustain a sense of inner tranquility in the face of physical uncertainties. To remain psychologically fit while physically in pain requires that the patient come to believe that his/her personal worth goes beyond his/her physical limitations. The development of such a belief can give chronically-ill patients develop a more hopeful and positive approach to their illness. In other words, a chronically-ill patient needs to be self-empowered in order to truly adapt to his/her illness and cope with the continuous pain and fatigue inherent in the disease. Often by developing peace, hope, and inner joy, the patient is better able to cope with some of his/her physical disabilities and weaknesses.

Fear can paralyze a chronically-ill patient in other ways too. Many chronically-ill patients are afraid of the future and what it may hold. Chronic illness is not something that can be controlled by anyone. However, worrying about which disabilities *may* occur in the future is a waste of time and precious energy. Thus, it is essential for a chronically-ill patient to face his/her illness with equanimity and live each day as fully as possible, despite his/her pain and fatigue. This can be hard to achieve at first but it is a mindset worth developing.

For example, if a chronically-ill patient is having a difficult day, (s)he should be extra kind to him/herself by taking ample rest periods during the day. In addition, the chronically-ill patient should not let bad days get him/her down but instead take steps to cope with the symptoms and fatigue during each part of the day. If a chronically-ill patient can develop and maintain such a positive attitude over time, (s)he will be better cope with his/her disabilities and fatigue.

# Gaining Control Over a Chronic Illness

There are *at least* four things that a chronically-ill patient can feasibly do to feel more in control of his/her illness. First, the patient could educate him/herself about the chronic illness she is living with. Knowledge is power and the more a chronically-ill patient can learn about his/her illness, the better (s)he will be able to cope with it. Every chronic illness requires a patient to learn how to adapt to his/her *version* of the disease. This is because every chronic illness is patient-specific and must be uniquely accommodated by physicians.

Second, patients should learn how to manage the unique challenges which are inherent in their own personal situation. It can be difficult for a newly diagnosed chronically-ill patient to moderate his/her life so that (s)he can positively live and cope with his/her illness. First and foremost, the patient must *realize* and *accept* that his/her life will never be the same again. The patient will always have to revise his/her actions, behaviours, energy levels, and especially lifestyle, to accommodate the chronic illness. There are quite a few different self-management techniques that a chronically-ill patient can try to ease pain and fatigue, such as using assistive devices, practising relaxation techniques, and putting certain stress-reducing mechanisms in place. I will discuss these mechanisms in more detail later on in the book.

Third, a chronically-ill patient should try not to be defined by her illness. Otherwise, the patient may develop low self-esteem because of the continuous nature of the pain and disability (s)he experiences, and the inability to do what (s)he previously did with ease. It can be difficult for a patient to feel positive and joyful under these circumstances. This negative outlook can frame a patient's life and make it much harder for the patient to cope with his/her disease over time. If chronically-ill patients develop low self-esteem, they can experience even more pain, and feel unable to cope with the physical symptoms and psychological ramifications of their illness.

One of the reasons why the way a patient feels about herself affects pain and disability is because if she feels down and has low self-esteem, she won't be able to effectively take control of the symptoms and disabilities related to her disabilities. Low self-esteem weakens the patient's ability to cope and effectively live with the illness over time. The patient must remember that she is still the person she is, and nothing changed about the essence of who she is. The only thing that has changed is his/her physical condition because of the onset of chronic illness.

Thus, it is essential for chronically-ill patients to realize that they should not be overcritical towards themselves regardless of their disabilities. Instead, a chronically-ill patient should realize that (s)he is not his/her illness. The chronically-ill patient should strive to develop positive self-esteem by being hopeful in the face of physical obstacles and the basic challenges of living with disabilities, to develop a positive self-image, and to realize that everyone has a basic right to live a peaceful and happy life, especially people with a chronic illness. But only we can bring this positive state of well-being about for ourselves.

Lastly, a chronically-ill patient should learn how to positively adapt to the physical and psychological symptoms of his/her illness. This is probably the most difficult part of coping with a chronic illness. When a patient is diagnosed with a chronic illness, (s)he won't be able to do the things which (s)he used to. Because of this, the patient may feel frustrated and angry. But by learning to live with the illness and developing a positive attitude towards it, a patient can still develop a wholesome quality of life that is enjoyable.

# Conclusion

In this chapter, I examined the nature of chronic illness and how chronically-ill patients can ensure that they do their part to take care of themselves. One major theme of this book highlights the unpredictable nature of illness for medical practice and how physicians can come to terms with it. Chronic-illness is patient-specific and because of this, different patients will cope with the disease in a very different manner, depending on their personality, stress levels, and life situation. One major purpose of this chapter is to show physicians the importance of encouraging chronically-ill patients to take control of their lives, despite their disabilities. A chronically-ill patient doesn't have to simply wait for things to get worse before (s)he learns how to positively cope with his/her illness. Instead, the patient must learn to be hopeful in order to preserve his/her self-esteem and quality of life. As I will show in Part II of this book, with practice and discipline, patients can reframe their lives in this positive way.

# Chapter 3

## Patient-Related Problems when Dealing with a Chronic Illness

### Introduction

Many chronically-ill patients find it difficult to be proactive about different aspects of their lives, especially when they are first diagnosed with the illness. Patients feel out of control and angry. After the diagnosis, many chronically-ill patients live in what is regarded as *the crisis stage*. During this stage, the patient often feels hopeless and frightened about the future, making it difficult for him/her to effectively take control of his/her life.

To deal the physical symptoms and control the psychological ramifications of the chronic illness, the patient must: (1) comply with the treatments prescribed by the physician and other medical specialists; (2) accept the illness and not be in denial about it; (3) take steps to gain control over the symptoms of the illness; (4) honestly deal with the psychological ramifications of the illness; and (5) develop self-management techniques to help cope with the effects of the illness as effectively as possible. By following these steps, chronically-ill patients will be living most successfully with a chronic illness. I will explain each of these components in more detail below.

### 1.

Chronically-ill patients should comply with all the treatments that the physician and other health experts prescribe. This can be a murky area for many chronically-ill patients because some individuals don't really understand the purpose of some of the treatments prescribed. For the treatments and medications to be helpful, however, patients MUST take their medications EXACTLY as prescribed by the physician. Also, if the physician prescribes other treatments, such as physiotherapy to ease pain and increase mobility, the patient must follow-through on the physician's advice. By precisely following the treatments prescribed by a patient's health care team, (s)he will be taking the necessary steps to manage the symptoms of his/her disease and gain control over the pain and disability (s)he experiences. Many patients, either intentionally or unintentionally, fail to follow a physician's verbal advice. This can be detrimental to a patient's success in effectively coping with her illness. Patients have to remember that their physicians are experts and therefore their advice should be followed to the letter.

# 2.

In addition, chronically-ill patients must accept their illness and decide to take concrete steps to cope with it so that their quality of life is not negatively impacted. Chronically-ill patients may be in denial about their illness, especially when they are first diagnosed, but this does not help their situation. Instead, chronically-ill patients should accept their chronic illness as an obstacle that must be dealt with directly at all times. Then, patients should move forward knowing that, although they can't change their overall diagnosis, they can control how they react to it by learning how to most effectively deal with the symptoms.

The worse thing a patient can do is to be in denial about his/her illness. Having a chronic illness can be an emotional roller coaster ride for many patients since they may not be able to move or live as they did at the onset of the illness or get nearly as much accomplished. Thus, chronically-ill patients will have to curb their previous activities and pace themselves in order not to suffer from overwhelming amounts of pain and fatigue. Chronic illness can zap a patient's overall physical and psychological vitality. However, chronically-ill patients can take steps to live a good quality of life by reprioritizing their daily activities and pacing themselves.

# 3.

Further, chronically-ill patients can gain control over their symptoms by planning ahead for activities that take a great deal of energy. For instance, it is natural for a chronically-ill patient to feel angry after realizing that (s)he no longer has as much energy to do the same things as (s)he used to. This is especially the case if the patient is still very young or merely middle aged. A patient should try to manage his/her busier days by planning ahead so that (s)he doesn't become totally exhausted and experience extreme pain as a result. Or, if a patient has a dinner party coming up, (s)he should start preparing for the event a few weeks ahead of time. By pacing and taking frequent breaks, the patient can better control the symptoms of the chronic illness.

Second, a chronically-ill patient can gain control over the symptoms of his/her illness by turning negative thoughts about the illness and how she feels into positive ones. An individual should incorporate small changes into his/her life so that they will lessen his/her pain and fatigue levels over time. This can improve the quality of the individual's life over time as well. For instance, if carrying heavy loads causes pain, the person should consider getting a pull wagon on wheels to distribute the load. Or, if the patient's pain medication causes negative side effects, she should try taking the medication before going to bed. This will help the patient to more effectively cope with the symptoms of his/her disease.

Third, the patient should learn problem-solving techniques to help resolve some of his/her daily pains, and discomforts. One of the first steps is for the chronically-ill patient to determine what his/her problems are, brainstorm solutions, and try one solution for two weeks to see if it helps improve pain and disability levels. This will ensure that the patient gains more self-control over his/her illness. There are solutions to most of a chronically-ill patient's problems if (s)he only has to take the motivation to discover them with an open and hopeful mind.

# 4.

Chronically-ill patients often suffer from bouts of depression, anxiety, or even anger. Sadly, it is as normal for the chronically-ill patient to experience depression as having physical disabilities. Therefore, it is important for patients to develop proper coping mechanisms for bad days. This way, patients wouldn't be negatively impacted by different forms of psychological distress that is related to their illness. A chronically-ill patient can often become quite overwhelmed on many different levels. That feeling usually occurs when the patient isn't able to take care of him/herself as (s)he used to. There are quite a few things patients can do to feel more in control of their chronic illness.

First, chronically-ill patients should be in habitual contact with others. It can be especially difficult for patients to deal with their pain if they live in isolation since they usually require a lot of support, ideally from various sources. Chronically-ill patients should join a support group of individuals who are experiencing similar daily difficulties. There is no better feeling than knowing that the individual is not alone in his/her predicament.

There are many workshops and online forums which are meant to give the chronically-ill patient the opportunity to meet other people who are suffering from similar ailments. Some of these workshops and forums are offered at the local hospital, YMCA or Community Care Access Center. Look for a list of these local events in your local newspaper or public bulletin boards in the library. Many chronically-ill patients are not as motivated as they should be to help themselves. However, with a bit of encouragement from others, we can all learn to take back our lives and not be defined by the disease.

Second, chronically-ill patients should deepen personal relationships with family members. Some families are not very understanding or compassionate about the chronically-ill patient's plight because of a fundamental lack of understanding of how difficult it is to always be in pain and experience disability. Thus, it is important for patients to open lines of communication with their family members. Sometimes, a chronic illness can bring family members closer. In addition, chronically-ill patients should openly talk about their symptoms and difficulties with their spouse. It is important for the spouse to take the time to show the person plagued with a chronic illness extra care and empathy. Further, patients should be able to speak openly about how they feel with their family without feeling harshly judged or criticized. This often occurs in families and it could add to the anxiety of living with the disease.

In addition, chronically-ill patients should delegate tasks when they need it to do so. Many chronically-ill patients feel ashamed to ask for help because they feel helpless when they do. Individuals believe that they should do everything they used to do before becoming chronically-ill. But this expectation isn't realistic to expect because chronic illnesses can be very physically debilitating. And much of the success in living with a chronic illness depends on adapting and modifying what and how an individual accommodates to his/her *new* reality. Thus, one important part of coping with a chronic condition is delegating tasks to others. This can ease the patient's pain and help break the pain cycle.

# 5.

A chronically-ill patient could alleviate some of the psychological and physical aspects of illness by practising several important self-management techniques. I will list four of the most important ones below. However, I will say more about self-management in the last chapter. First, exercise can help a chronically-ill patient feel more flexible and mobile. Since most of us have learned to dislike the word *exercise*, perhaps calling it movement or physical activity is better. Whatever we decide to call it isn't important. However, it is very important for patients to do *some form of physical activity* at least 20 to 30 minutes a day, three to four times a week in order to feel healthy, more mobile, and happy. In addition, exercise can help chronically-ill patients sleep better. So, exercise is a definite benefit to the patient.

Second, the chronically-ill patient should develop a positive attitude towards life by developing a sense of humour, not taking life too seriously, celebrating special moments, and having hope that everything will turn out for the best. It isn't always easy for a patient to develop such a positive attitude when (s)he is in constant pain. Life for a chronically-ill patient can be an uphill battle. However, by developing a positive mindset, even difficult days could be made easier.

Third, chronically-ill patients should meditate daily. Meditation can be as simple as closing your eyes and shutting out the world around you while relaxing your mind and soul. This can create a sense of peace and serenity which can be very comforting for chronically-ill patients. Having a regular meditation practice can also help chronically-ill patients come to terms with how they feel about themselves and their disabilities. By practising meditation once or twice a day, for even as little as five to ten minutes at a time for a few weeks, the chronically-ill patient can ease tension and become much more relaxed and experience less pain.

Fourth, chronically-ill patients should practice extreme self-care. To do so, patients must schedule time for themselves every day. They should try to choose things they enjoy doing and spend time doing them. Extreme self-care is the practice of going to great lengths to take care of one's mind, body, and soul. Further, extreme self-care means that the patient must put him/herself first and take care of his/her needs for an extended period of time. Some self-care activities could include taking a warm bubble bath, reading, lying down or taking a quiet walk. The benefits of extreme self-care are usually long-lasting for the chronically-ill patient.

By following these self-management techniques, chronically-ill patients can live much more balanced and happy lives. It is hard to overestimate the fact that it is hard to live with a chronic illness. However, there's so much that patients can do to help themselves cope with their illness and disability. Chronically-ill patients can take small baby steps to make their lives easier. By following the steps outlined in this chapter, chronically-ill patients can make their lives more than just an uphill battle. Patients can learn how to thrive and live their best life, despite their chronic condition.

# Chapter 4

---

# Physician-Related Problems when Dealing with a Chronic Illness

## Introduction

Most diagnosis and treatments in medical practice are measured by some scientific evidence. Yet, chronic illness doesn't lend itself to such a scientific formulation of treatment options. Because of this, physicians may find it difficult to prescribe treatments that involve measurable kinds of assessments since there is no guarantee that these treatments and medications will actually help a chronically-ill patient. But more than that, monitoring the progress of such treatments can be especially difficult too. Such unpredictable treatment results can frustrate the physician, given the fairly predictable nature of medical practice, making it difficult for him/her to know if (s)he is really helping the patient in any significant way. The unpredictable nature of caring for a chronically-ill patient is very different in nature from acutely-ill patients in that there are no one-size-fits-all cures to alleviate the symptoms of the illness.

Thus, the process of treating a chronically-ill patient can be time consuming and especially costly for several reasons. First, chronically-ill patients must be booked for longer appointment times because their symptoms are not always clear cut. The physician may also come to realize that, for some patients, the symptoms can be psychosomatic, further complicating the clinical encounter. In addition, some chronically-ill patients may be afraid that they are seriously-ill, or they may be worried that their disabilities will get worse as time goes on. Sadly, chronic illnesses don't miraculously get better. Rather, the physical disabilities involved in a chronic illness usually get worse over time. This can negatively affect the overall morale of the clinical encounter. It can also make it difficult for the chronically-ill patient to become proactive when living with the illness because of how hopeless she feels.

Second, it may be difficult for the physician to effectively probe into the causes of the chronic illness because they are not always straightforward. The physician usually has to ask questions about the patient's family background and life circumstances. This can take time, effort, and a lot of detective work. It can be hampered by the vague descriptions of the patient's symptoms. Many times, they defy accurate description and measurement. Over time, through a lot of investigation, the physician will discover some of the underlying causes of the illness, such as undue stress or an unhealthy lifestyle.

Third, chronic illness is usually unobservable and the symptoms are largely immeasurable. Most chronically-ill patients don't have many outward physical manifestations of disability. They mostly look like normal and healthy people. The difficulty with experiencing unobservable symptoms is that the physician cannot always get an accurate sense of the pain, disability, and discomfort that the patient is experiencing just through a physical examination. In addition, the pain is often subjective and patient-specific, adding to the ambiguity of providing adequate treatment options.

For instance, having a chronic illness is not like having a broken leg that requires surgery or treatment. Once the leg is healed, the pain disappears and the patient can resume his/her life. For most chronically-ill patients, the pain lingers for many months, years or even a lifetime. In addition, most times, chronically-ill patients have a difficult time precisely describing their pain or pointing to where it is located. Sometimes, the pain experienced seems to be all over the body. There is also very little that a physician can prescribe to substantially help the patient's overall pain levels or quality of life. In other words, there is no *magic bullet* to alleviate pain and suffering once and for all. This can be especially frustrating for the patient.

Thus, there are very few evidence-based guidelines that physicians can rely on to treat chronically-ill patients. For instance, since a patient's pain levels are largely patient-specific, it is difficult for the physician to accurately assess how much pain a patient is really experiencing at any given time. Pain cannot be observed. Instead, physicians have to rely on the patient's subjective report of pain. Sometimes, physicians may treat chronic pain in a sceptical manner which can further complicate the interaction with chronically-ill patients since, if trust is undermined in any way, the physician–patient relationship will be undermined. As I'll show in Part II of the book, without developing trust, an open and honest relationship cannot be developed between physician and patient. A physician's medical training is very systematic and measurable which can make it more difficult for him/her to clearly understand the elusive symptoms described by the patient.

To remedy this situation, I believe that the physician needs to rely on another paradigm of medical care to treat chronically-ill patients, one that is based on the qualitative aspects of medical care. This is where the patient-centered approach outlined in Part II is not only relevant but necessary. The four conditions of the patient-centered approach should facilitate the physician-patient encounter and make it more wholesome and meaningful both for the patient and physician. I will briefly outline the four conditions below.

# The Four Conditions of the Patient-Centered Approach

The patient-centered approach gives the patient priority in a medical interaction. It is an approach that is empathic to a patient's concerns and overall well-being. Because this approach is patient-based, it is much less measurable and much more subjective than the typical clinical encounter. And this is to be expected when treating chronically-ill patients. The nature of chronic illness is such that physicians must treat the particular patient more than the disease itself. Chronic illness makes patients vulnerable and uncertain, and physicians must try to address such immeasurable concerns during the clinical encounter.

The four conditions of the patient-centered approach to be discussed in Part II highlight these subjective concerns. The four principles focus on developing a humane, empathic, open, honest, and trusting relationship with a patient so that she can make rational decisions for or against treatment and for the physician to come to terms with the unpredictable nature of chronic illness. Here is a brief synopsis of the four conditions of the patient-centered approach for the chronically-ill to be discussed in more detail in the next four chapters of the book.

The first condition requires that the physician engage in empathic communication with the patient. This ultimately requires that the physician understand the patient and develop a trusting relationship with him/her. Trust can help physicians to mend the communication gaps that may exist between themselves and their patients. To develop trust, the patient should feel comfortable to openly disclose any of his/her symptoms to the physician, and the physician should seek to understand the patient's predicament, despite the fact some of the symptoms may defy accurate measurement. Sometimes, a patient's feelings are all that physicians have to go on to make a diagnosis.

The second condition encourages physicians to understand their patients. Understanding is one of the most important principles which physicians can display to chronically-ill patients during the clinical encounter. The nature of chronic illness is such that it is difficult for the patient to always feel supported and cared for due to the constant pain and discomfort she feels. Some chronically-ill patients will develop low self-esteem because they are unable to perform the activities they used to do. Other chronically-ill patients may even become depressed and feel hopeless. Because of the chronically-ill patient's vulnerabilities, it is essential for the physician to try and *imagine what it would be like* to experience constant pain and fatigue that is similar to what the patient is always feeling. Then the physician can more effectively help the patient.

The third condition highlights the importance of shared or mutual decision-making between physician and patient. Shared decision-making occurs when the physician, along with the patient, tries to make a mutual decision about a treatment option or surgery. It can be difficult for chronically-ill patients to make rational decisions on their own. Many times, chronically-ill patients will make biased decisions for or against a treatment based on subjective feelings. It is, therefore, important for the physician to *guide* such patients into much more rational and unbiased decisions by helping them to realize that certain treatments and/or surgeries can make the quality of their lives so much better. Many chronically-ill patients may frame the benefits of treatments in terms of the drawbacks involved instead of the benefits that may ensue. This can hinder the patient from making rational decisions about their treatment options which may help him/her feel less pain in the long run.

The fourth condition encourages the physician and patient to develop an effective relationship so that they can talk openly to each other during the clinical encounter. It is especially important for physicians who treat chronically-ill patients to develop an open and honest relationship. To do so, the physician must spend a considerable amount of time attentively listening to the patient in order to understand how the patient is coping, given the symptoms of his/her chronic illness. It's never easy to develop an open, honest relationship with a patient who may be depressed, especially when the physician knows that (s)he can never completely alleviate the patient's pain and discomfort. The nature of medical practice is such that physicians are used to treating patients and alleviating pain. And for most patients, except the chronically-ill, this is indeed possible. However, the chronically-ill patient is a different kind of patient and presents a distinct set of challenges for the physician.

In practicing these four conditions, the physician and patient will be accepting the unpredictable nature of the patient's symptoms. Because of this, a chronically-ill patient's treatments may also be unpredictable, with no clear-cut answers. Therefore, the clinical encounter for a chronically-ill patient is very different than for acute care patients. By realizing this, the physician should not expect predictable results when treating chronically ill patients. Instead, physicians must realize that the chronically-ill patient's treatments will not always work. This underlies the unpredictable nature of medical practice when treating the chronically-ill.

# Conclusion

Thus, physicians must develop a unique patient-centered approach for each chronically-ill patient. This will help physicians to feel less frustrated and more accepting of the unpredictable nature of medical care that must be administered for chronically-ill patients. In Part II, I will examine these four conditions of the patient-centered approach for the chronically-ill patient in detail. I will argue that once these conditions are met by physicians, they will be able to treat chronically-ill patients in a humane manner. In addition, the patient-centered approach will help physicians develop a type of medical care that is best suited to the chronically-ill patient.

# Part II

# Chapter 5

## Empathic Physician–Patient Communication

### Introduction

The first condition of the patient-centered approach is empathic physician-patient communication. An important part of the patient-centered approach is for the physician to learn how to communicate clearly and compassionately with the patient about his/her medical concerns. Every chronically-ill patient will have unique challenges to cope with because of his/her illness. It is, therefore, important for physicians to try and make patients feel at ease as much as possible. Patients must be encouraged to take charge of their health because of the nature of their illness. So, *empathic physician–patient communication* is required to bring about humane health because it is one important aspect of caring for a chronically-ill patient. The patient-centered approach makes the patient's concerns a top priority in every medical encounter. This approach can help a patient feel empowered and encouraged at a time when (s)he may feel vulnerable, fearful, anxious, miserable, and perhaps even uncertain.

There are three dimensions of empathic communication. These are as follows:

1. Open and honest discussion of symptoms;
2. A discussion of the patient's fears surrounding increased disability; and
3. Empathy with the patient's predicament.

Each of these three dimensions of communication will be especially beneficial in helping the chronically-ill patient to more readily accept and deal with his/her illness. These dimensions can also help the patient overcome the overwhelming frustration and anxiety of living with a chronic condition.

## Developing Open, Honest Communication

When the patient is diagnosed with a chronic illness, such as arthritis, the physician should determine the most effective way to communicate with the patient about that illness based on that patient's specific needs. Each patient's needs are different and unique. The medical encounter should be such that the patient feels comfortable enough to ask questions and seek clarifications about treatments and other medical interventions. In addition, the physician should carefully listen to a patient's avowals of pain and discomfort. The physician may also have to try to fill in some grey areas in the discussion, with the patient's help. Grey areas occur when the patient is unable to clearly explain his/her symptoms or the frequency of them. The physician should not negatively judge a patient's questions and categorize them as trivial. Every question is acceptable because it reveals that patient's *unique* concerns and worries about the nature of the illness and how it impacts his/her life.

There are two central components of empathic communication, *openness* and *honesty*, both of which are similar and yet distinct to a certain degree. *Openness* and *honesty* are necessary when the physician discusses how the patient can best cope with the chronic illness. Many psychologists and philosophers categorize *openness* as an aspect of *honesty*. However, the two concepts don't mean the same thing and should be separated in order to clearly distinguish between them during a clinical encounter.

On the one hand, *Openness* typically has a psychological and subjective function in communication while *honesty* has a much more objective function. When a physician is *open* with the chronically-ill patient, (s)he allows a patient to express any emotions and fears that patient might experience about the chronic illness. On the other hand, when a physician is *honest*, (s)he usually discusses how an illness and disability will affect a patient's life.

In addition, the physician can express *openness* towards the patient through gestures and body language. Therefore, *honesty* also has an objective component. To be fully honest with the patient, the physician should disclose the results of his/her diagnosis in detail, without withholding any aspect of it. For instance, after running a few X-rays, the physician may discover that the patient has disability or inflammation in other parts of the body. It is important for the physician to disclose this fact to the patient. Arthritis can present a lot of puzzling physical manifestations for arthritis patients, such as nodes and lumps. These should also be discussed by the physician.

The subjective aspect of *openness* is that the physician must provide the patient with a sufficient amount of time to decide whether or not to undergo a medical procedure, after the initial communication. This is especially the case for invasive treatments such as knee replacement operations or back surgery. The physician may also want to meet with the patient a few days or a week after the initial disclosure to discuss any other matters that have surfaced and answer any further questions. Each chronically-ill patient has a unique way of coping with the diagnosis and treatment. Thus, the physician should determine how much consultation time is necessary for each patient in order for that patient to feel secure and encouraged.

One way to convey an *open* attitude is for the physician to sit close to the patient when disclosing the diagnosis so that the physician can comfort the patient, if need be. This gesture usually helps to show a sense of emotional openness and comfort to the patient. Another way to be open towards the patient is for the physician to speak in a low, comforting tone by using empathic and reassuring language when discussing the illness such as:

*"I know this must be hard for you to cope with";*
*"It must be hard to live with so much pain all the time";*
*"It must be hard to be so young and yet in so much pain";*
    *And so on . . .*

This will help the patient feel understood and encourage him/her to carry on, despite the patient's pain and suffering which the chronic illness poses on a daily basis.

# Discussion of the Patient's Fears Surrounding Disabilities

After the disclosure of diagnosis and possible treatment options, the physician must also leave a sufficient amount of time to discuss the patient's fears about the future. A patient diagnosed with chronic illness is usually plagued with all kinds of fears and uncertainties. Most times, family members are not available, either physically or psychologically, to talk openly with the patient. Also, many families do not often talk about their deepest concerns openly. So, the patient may become secretive and refrain from telling the family members the whole truth about his/her disabilities until (s)he absolutely has to.

Another way the physician could encourage the chronically-ill patient to talk about his/her fears is by asking open-ended questions such as: *How have you felt since the diagnosis? Are you scared about the future? Can you keep working part-time? Which hobbies do you want to keep doing, despite the pain and fatigue? Do you still feel a lot of pain? Does your pain medication help alleviate the pain so that you can function properly and work?* This type of probing process is especially important for patients who may have a difficult time effectively communicating with the physician. Some patients don't know where to start or how to voice their concerns. Many patients haven't spoken to anyone about their concerns and difficulties for years, so they don't even know how to effectively communicate about them in any kind of clear manner. By asking open-ended questions, the physician will engage the patient and hopefully make it easier for him/her to openly discuss his/her fears.

# Empathy with a Patient's Predicament

Empathy is another important feature of effective communication. Many times, the patient may feel insufficiently cared for because the physician may appear to be unintentionally uncompassionate or uncaring. Empathy shows a chronically-ill patient that the physician genuinely cares about his/her medical predicament. In the process of empathic listening, a physician should listen carefully to the patient's questions and concerns. The physician must also try to understand the patient's feelings, determine the meaning of the patient's fears, and encourage the patient to reframe his/her negative attitudes towards the chronic illness. In other words, an empathic physician must sense, intuit, and empathize with a patient's predicament as much as possible. To show empathy, the physician should feel genuinely sorry for the patient's situation and do everything medically possible to help the patient. Sympathy alone is insufficient to help a patient cope with the effects of a chronic condition since sympathy merely involves feeling sorry for the patient. Instead, empathy shows the patient that the physician genuinely cares about his/her struggles and can put him/herself in the patient's shoes.

Empathy is, therefore, essential to bring about a humanistic, patient-centered encounter between physician and patient. The physician should imagine what it would be like to experience the pain and disability the patient feels. Empathy is best understood as a tool that will assist in understanding the patient's predicament—not merely the feelings of communion or fellow-feeling with the other person, as would be the case with a sympathetic response to the patient.

The traditional paradigm of medical practice views chronic illness as a disease that could be *fixed* using various kinds of treatment and/or surgery. In a strictly medical assessment, a diseased state is an entity that can be separated from the patient experiencing the illness. For the chronically-ill patient, a medical assessment has to be combined with the patient-centered approach to best treat a chronically-ill patient. Any chronic illness negatively impacts the quality of a patient's life on a daily basis. The difference between a strictly medical conceptualization of chronic illness as a disease and the patient's interpretation as a lived experience of the illness which affects every aspect of his/her life, highlights the reason why the patient and physician may find it so difficult to effectively communicate with one another about his/her physical and especially psychophysical struggles. The physician's approach is mostly objective while the patient's is mostly subjective. The patient-centered approach advocated in this book tries to soften this dichotomy between the subjective and objective approaches to illness by encouraging the physician to show more empathy and a subjective, patient-centered element into every encounter with a chronically-ill patient.

# Conclusion

Thus, empathic communication is the foundation for achieving patient-centered care for the chronically-ill. Without empathic communication not only will the physician–patient relationship be hampered but the interaction between the two will be detached and impersonal. One important condition of a patient-centered approach is that a chronically-ill patient requires an empathic encounter between physician and patient to most effectively deal with the symptoms of the disease. This will lay the foundation of trust and acceptance that is necessary for the physician to help the patient effectively cope with the illness. In addition, an empathic encounter is a foundational element of the three other conditions of the patient-centered approach to be discussed in the chapters that follow.

# Chapter 6

# Effective Physician–Patient Understanding

The second condition of the patient-centered approach is effective physician–patient understanding during the clinical encounter. Understanding requires a multi-staged analysis by the physician to determine that the patient indeed understands all the information disclosed about the diagnosis and prognosis and that she can make a rational decision about the best course of treatment, given her chronic illness. In this chapter, I will outline this process, detailing some of the difficulties inherent in shared understanding.

Chronically-ill patients are in a category of their own. They are unlike any other patient that the physician will treat. One important condition of a patient-centered approach to chronic care is to ensure that the physician fully understands the patient's difficulties and disabilities. This isn't always easy to achieve, given the ambiguities of chronic illness and the difficulty of getting a clear sense of the patient's needs. This can take a lot of time for the physician to achieve. But by trying to understand the patient's concerns, the physician can bring about a patient-centered approach to treating his/her patient.

## Bringing About Effective Understanding

An effective disclosure of a diagnosis requires that the patient understands the diagnosis, prognosis, and treatments outlined by the physician. Generally, an effective disclosure is an exchange between two individuals that has the overriding purpose of presenting information clearly and assisting understanding. Understanding may be characterized as the physician's assimilation of the information about a patient's illness and life situation and his/her understanding of the treatment options available. The criteria for understanding the disclosure of a diagnosis are complex since these involve psychological and intellectual idiosyncrasies which are unique to each patient. Each patient's degree and level of understanding must be intuitively assessed by the physician.

Several factors may be instrumental in ensuring that a medical disclosure is properly understood by the patient. First, according to the patient-centered model, a chronically-ill patient must *substantially* understand the diagnosis, prognosis, and communication about the treatments available to him/herself. A substantial amount of information is usually disclosed by the physician about the possible treatments available to the patient. Some of the types of medical information that may be disclosed include the diagnosis, all the risks and benefits for each treatment, the side effects for each treatment, and a ranking of the benefits of each treatment.

Second, each of these factors requires a detailed analysis. To make this information clear, the physician should schedule some extra time for the patient to process the information. This is especially the case for ranking the benefits of each treatment since the assessment usually requires an analysis and prioritization of the treatments available. This process requires that the patient can properly assimilate all the information disclosed. Understanding this information can be a complex process, depending on the patient's ability to understand such information when it is explained by the physician.

## The Three Conditions of Effective Understanding

Thus, as you can see, understanding between physician and patient is quite a complicated process. It involves clear understanding and shared nuances that only the patient can provide. In this section, I will outline and discuss the three conditions of understanding. These are: (1) Shared understanding; (2) Determining the relevancy of information disclosed; and (3) Using medical jargon sparingly.

## Shared Understanding

There is an important difference between *shared understanding* and *ordinary understanding*. *Shared understanding* is based on a reciprocal understanding between the physician and patient. *Ordinary understanding,* on the other hand, merely consists of communicating the facts, and the risks and benefits for each treatment, without attempting to take the patient's personal needs, values, and situation into consideration. It is insufficient for the physician to simply communicate the raw facts and the risks and benefits of the treatments to the patient since the treatments will feel impersonal to the particular chronically-ill patient. Instead, the physician must personalize how she presents the treatments and their risks.

*Shared understanding* takes place when the physician understands the details of the patient's values, goals, beliefs, and life plans in relation to her illness. The physician then must operate within certain medical constraints which are, in effect, beyond his/her control. Both the physician and patient must, therefore, comprehend each other in a subjective, person-to-person manner, which allows each of them to openly and honestly communicate without manipulation or disingenuousness. The chronically-ill patient's feelings of grief and vulnerability can be greatly eased with such a shared understanding.

## Determining the Relevancy of Information Disclosed

Initially, the physician must reveal all the treatments available, without prioritizing them so that the *relevancy of the information disclosed* can be determined by the physician and patient. Then both the patient and physician should eliminate the irrelevant treatments, evaluating the remaining alternatives in greater detail. It should never merely be the physician's sole responsibility to decide which treatments are relevant to a particular chronically-ill patient. Relevancy is difficult to establish right away because it is usually unique to the patient and his/her psychological state. The unique personal and psychological manifestations of a chronic illness are difficult to unravel without communicating with the patient at length. Ensuring that a chronically-ill patient is included in the process of choosing the relevant treatments invites that patient into the decision-making process for treating his/her own illness. This, in turn, ensures that the patient feels more in control of his/her chronic illness. This kind of shared decision-making also ensures that the patient is competent to decide which treatments are best to schedule in the near future and which to forgo.

## Using Medical Jargon Sparingly

*If the treatments are disclosed to the patient using strictly medical terminology*, (s)he will not be able to fully understand the disclosure. Medical terminology is usually considered to be a convenient short-hand; but when communicating with a patient, these treatments should be translated into ordinary language so that the patient is able to understand. The patient has no medical training, and although most patients are better informed about health matters today than a few decades ago, technical medical jargon can still make it impossible for most patients to effectively understand the disclosure. Thus, the physician should be extremely careful about how much medical jargon she uses when disclosing information about the treatments available.

Different patients have different capacities for understanding. Some patients are more informed and better able to understand physicians. Other patients have a difficult time understanding the treatments disclosed by the physician. The degree of difficulty in understanding can depend on many different factors. Some of these are as follows: (a) Levels of education; (b) Capacities for reflectiveness; and (c) Psychological factors, such as (i) relentless pain; (ii) feelings of hopelessness and depression; and (iii) denial.

### *Levels of Education*

Differing levels of education affect how, or even whether, a patient will grasp and understand the medical information disclosed by the physician. In addition, there will be a difference in how long a patient takes to comprehend the medical information provided by the physician. Chronically-ill patients with secondary and post-secondary education do not pose as serious a problem for physicians as patients who lack secondary education. This latter group of patients make the practice of shared understanding especially difficult to bring about. This is because they can't process the information adequately or understand what is being disclosed. This adds to the difficulty of treating such patients because being clear and concise isn't really helpful. They pose special problems that are beyond the scope of this book.

## *Capacities for Reflectiveness*

Differing levels of patient reflectiveness and comprehension could also affect a patient's understanding of the alternatives disclosed. It is pretty easy for a physician to determine whether or not a chronically-ill patient is sufficiently reflective so that (s)he will not make hasty decisions about medical treatments. Reflective patients usually insist on having an adequate amount of time to think about the treatments, ask questions about important aspects of the treatment and their illness that they don't understand, and decide whether or not to start a particular treatment on the basis of their values, goals, and life plans. If the patient asks such questions, she is reflective.

Although most patients seem to be sufficiently reflective, except perhaps for the uneducated, the quality and degree of a patient's reflective capacity may still vary substantially. Some patients may be reflective enough to think about the treatments disclosed by the physician, but may still decide to undergo a treatment hastily, not taking the necessary time to carefully reflect on the treatments and their side effects. Some of these patients usually fail to have a coherent set of values, goals, and life plans available for them to make a proper, autonomous choice about a medical treatment. Yet other patients are quite unreflective. In this case, the physician must *guide* an unreflective patient's thinking in an unbiased manner such that (s)he can make a proper decision for or against treatment.

## *Psychological Factors*

Three psychological factors can influence a patient's understanding. These are: (i) relentless pain and fatigue; and (ii) feelings of hopelessness and depression; and (iii) denial.

### Relentless Pain and Fatigue

*Relentless pain and fatigue* can affect a chronically-ill patient's capacity to understand the information about the treatments disclosed by the physician. When a chronically-ill patient is in constant pain, (s)he may not be able to concentrate properly. The chronically-ill patient usually desires to have his/her pain lessened as soon as possible. Therefore, such patients may 'frame' treatment solutions hastily because of their pain and discomfort levels. Upon recognition of such difficulties, physicians should take steps to *guide* a chronically-ill patient's thinking so that (s)he chooses the most appropriate treatments. In this way, the patient may be able to *step back* from his/her pain for a short time, and make a decision that is based on an objective understanding of all the treatments available.

## Feelings of Hopelessness and Depression

*Feelings of hopelessness and depression* may also be detrimental to a chronically-ill patient's capacity for understanding the treatments since such feelings can irrationally sway the patient towards inappropriate treatments. A chronically-ill patient does not have a *normal* life. Life is a constant uphill battle with no rhyme or reason sometimes. This can make rational unbiased decisions difficult to bring about.

Chronically-ill patients will *frame* the treatments differently from an acutely-ill patient. Acutely ill patients undergo treatment, take time to recover, and then resume their normal lives. However, a chronically-ill patient's reality is very different. The long-term nature of the illness may bias patients to *frame* decisions in terms of how hopeless they feel. The physician must keep this tendency towards biased decisions in mind since such decisions would be negative in nature.

## Denial

*Denial* is normal for a patient living with a chronic illness. Such patients are usually in denial about their illness and disability. Such an unrealistic mindset usually disrupts the mental composure of the patient. For some chronically-ill patients, the grief experienced is stronger and more intense than for other types of patients. This occurs for several reasons.

First, the chronically-ill patient may not have effective coping skills in place to deal with the symptoms of the fatigue and pain she experiences. Some patients may feel angry and depressed because of the continuous nature of pain and increased disability they experience. It may sometimes be necessary for the physician to recommend that the patient seeks counselling to learn how to best cope with the illness.

Second, the patient may not have a support system in place with people who are in a similar situation. Many families don't help chronically-ill patients and the unpredictable nature of the illness makes it especially difficult for the patient to be consistent with symptoms and fatigue levels. Family members may not believe the hardship the patient experiences because she *looks relatively healthy*. This can make chronically-ill patients feel even more alone and desperate at times. There's nothing worse than suffering in isolation. So, it is important for patients to seek support systems outside of the realm of their family. Contact your local chapter of the Arthritis Society or go online and seek out support groups. There are many opportunities out there; we just have to seek them out.

Third, the patient may be experiencing a difficult time because (s)he never expected to become chronically-ill. Chronic illness can be overwhelming to live with at first. Thus, it is important for a patient to take time to come to terms with the idea that she can no longer do as much as she did before. Unless chronically-ill patients grieve properly, they will be bitter and enraged as time goes on.

By taking these three psychological factors that can influence shared understanding into consideration, physicians can ensure that their patients have effectively understood the potential treatments. Without an understanding of the treatments, patients cannot make a rational decision about the treatment which is best for them.

# Conclusion

Chronically-ill patients offer new challenges for the physician, some of which may be difficult to overcome, given a physician's time constraints. There are no easy solutions for physicians. The difficulty is exacerbated by patients who aren't able to psychologically come to terms with their illness. By trying to ensure that patients understand their treatment options, physicians come closer to advocating patient-centered care, and when it comes to chronic care, that is very laudable indeed.

# Chapter 7

## Successful Decision-Making

The third condition of the patient-centered approach for the chronically-ill is shared decision-making. This type of decision-making is important since patients who suddenly become chronically-ill may not be able to make rational decisions about their future medical treatments on their own. It is, therefore, important that the patient make decisions about treatment options in conjunction with the physician. The physician's role is to *guide* the patient to make a rational decision about future treatments or medical procedures.

The difficulty with treating chronic illness is that a patient's decision-making capabilities may be biased because of uncertainty of the diagnosis. It is never easy for patients to hear the physician say that they have arthritis, diabetes, or some other chronic condition. We all hope that we'll always be healthy. However, this is an illusion since most of us will ultimately suffer from some type of chronic illness in our lives and we will have to make some important adjustments to our lives in order to cope and live the best life possible regardless.

In this chapter, I will focus on several overarching aspects of successful decision-making which underlie the patient-centered approach to medicine. The foundational components of successful decision-making are empathy and stepping back from a patient's negative attitudes towards the illness and treatment. But before I get ahead of myself, I'll discuss what constitutes a successful decision.

## Preliminary Characterization

For the purposes of this discussion, a successful decision is a rational and level-headed choice that is consistent with a patient's values, goals, beliefs and life plans, and which is not influenced by biases and prejudices which are irrelevant to the medical decision at hand. If a chronically-ill patient is on medication, in constant pain or experiencing extreme fatigue, his/her ability to think in a rational manner may be negatively affected. In such cases, the physician should either advise the patient to stop taking the medication before making an important medical decision, or *guide* the patient to ensure that his/her ultimate decision in favor or against treatment is rational.

According to the patient-centered model, any paternalistic form of influence on decision-making can violate a patient's cognitive capacity for making his/her own decisions about medical treatments. Physicians must, therefore, ensure that they are *guiding* the patient but not *prescribing* what they consider are the most beneficial treatments on the patient's behalf. To *guide* means to *think along with* the patient, and encourage him/her to deliberate rationally. This process is typically most effective when physicians keep asking the patient some specific questions about the treatments to ensure that (s)he has, in fact, fully understood them during the disclosure.

## The Three Dimensions of Rational Decision-Making

Chronically-ill patients usually experience some sort of continuous pain and fatigue for a prolonged period of time. Such patients may often been prescribed psychologically debilitating medications. The physician must devise special methodologies and procedures for making medical decisions with such a patient. It is obvious that physicians cannot ensure that a rational decision is made by each chronically-ill patient; however, if a patient has adequate self-knowledge, then the difficulty is manageable, and an informed consent about a treatment is still possible. Rational decisions cannot usually be made by chronically-ill patients who lack a substantial amount of self-knowledge.

There are three dimensions of rational decision-making: (1) Reflective deliberation; (2) Reflective Awareness; and (3) Empathic understanding.

## Reflective Deliberation

The successful achievement of reflective deliberation presupposes that the chronically-ill patient has rationally evaluated his/her choice of treatments and can make a rational decision on the basis of this self-evaluation. To rationally deliberate about a treatment, a patient must not allow emotional and/or psychological influences to enter into the decision-making process. This is a difficult stage of the deliberative process especially when a patient constantly feels depressed and uncertain because of the continuous pain and other kinds of distress that is involved in living with a chronic condition. There are many ways that physicians can *guide* such patients to be more reflective by ensuring that errors in reasoning do not occur. It can take time and patience for the physician to ensure that the chronically-ill patient makes a rational decision. However, this is one of important tasks for a physician since, without proper reflection, chronically-ill patients will not give an informed consent for treatment.

## Reflective Awareness

Reflective awareness is a process through which the mind becomes aware of its own operations. A more practical characterization is that reflective awareness is a process of examining our thinking processes, trying, for example, to determine how we derived our initial assessments. In order to achieve this, a chronically-ill patient must become introspective about his/her own thinking processes in order to retrace his/her initial deliberations. The terms *introspective*, *reflective*, and *deliberative* have distinctive meanings and should not be conflated or considered to mean more or less the same thing. In introspection, an individual must become aware of his/her own deliberative processes. Introspection is a process that makes it possible for a patient to become aware of her ordinary deliberations and reflective awareness. The evaluative stage of awareness, on the other hand, occurs at the reflective stage at which point the patient should make an assessment about his/her initial thinking processes in deriving her decision.

By practicing reflective awareness, a patient substantially increases his/her chances of making a rational decision about a medical treatment. It ensures that the patient will take the time to critically evaluate all the medical information disclosed by the physician and ensure that this decision is consistent with his/her values, goals, and life situation. This evaluative analysis takes a considerable amount of time and depends on the chronically-ill patient's ability to effectively reflect. Different patients have different capacities for this type of complex reflection, and not every person is equally reflective. In addition, continuous pain and suffering, and the side effects of certain medications can weaken a chronically-ill patient's reflective capacities. For patients who are negatively impacted by continuous pain, fatigue and medication, the reflective process should be attempted more than once to ensure their reflective evaluations are consistent and rational.

Thus, reflective awareness signifies more than the freedom to choose between alternative medical treatments. It requires that a chronically-ill patient makes a reflective choice that represents his/her deeply held beliefs and preferences. Chronically-ill patients are more than a bundle of individual behaviours; they are as capable of reflective awareness as other patients.

When a patient is reflectively aware, the physician won't have as much difficulty *guiding* a patient to make a proper choice of treatments. It will be possible to be much more confident in determining whether or not the chronically-ill patient has adequately understood the information disclosed, and whether or not his/her decision was influenced by other irrelevant considerations. The physician can do this by being attentive to the kinds of questions and clarifications that the chronically-ill patient asks. Most chronically-ill patients will make decisions that are consistent with the type of individuals that they are. For instance, if a chronically-ill patient is a Type-A personality, she will be more prone to making unreflective decisions; however, if a chronically-ill patient is peaceful and calm by nature before the diagnosis, she will probably make much more reflective decisions. These guidelines will help the physician determine which patients need to be *guided* to make a rational decision and which ones can make decisions on their own. Typically, if a patient exhibits reflective awareness, (s)he is able to make rational decisions in favour of a treatment on his/her own. However, patients who are not sufficiently reflective will need continuous guidance from the physician.

What if the physician, while disclosing the information about a medical treatment, recognizes that the patient lacks the skills for reflective deliberation and has decided on a treatment in a haphazard manner? Does the physician have a responsibility to probe further in order to enable the chronically-ill patient to comprehend all the information in a level-headed manner? On the patient-centered model, reflective deliberation is a central requirement of rational decision-making. Thus, the physician should take steps to ensure that a patient's decision is rational. The physician could help the patient by guiding and encouraging his/her thinking processes to a deeper and more rational reflection. While most chronically-ill patients can make rational decisions, to some degree, some patients will need a lot more guidance than others to make rational and reflective decisions about medical treatments.

## Empathic Understanding

One of the most important features of patient-centered health care is for the physician to ensure that the patient gives a proper consent for treatment. From a personal perspective, the chronically-ill patient may be depressed about his/her medical predicament. Empathy can help a physician detect many forms of psychological distress. If a patient's psychological distress goes untreated, it could result in experiencing premature despondency about her chronic condition. Thus, it is important for the physician to get to know the patient in order to determine whether or not different aspects of his/her chronic condition should be treated before (s)he makes a decision in favour of treatment. This is the interpersonal component of obtaining an informed consent for treatment. Through an empathic understanding of the patient's situation and by developing a relationship of mutual trust and respect, the physician will be able to determine whether or not (s)he should help the patient choose the best treatment. Below, I outline four *guidelines* which physicians should use to ensure that a chronically-ill patient gives an informed consent for treatment. As will be shown, empathy is the foundation for each of these *guidelines*.

First, a physician must gain a sufficient amount of knowledge about the patient, not only in terms of his/her medical history but also a sense of how she is uniquely coping with his/her chronic condition and how it is affecting her quality of life. This process involves becoming aware of the patient's values, desires, and long and short-term life goals. In addition, it is essential that the physician gain a sufficient amount of information about the patient's temperament, character traits, and attitudes. For instance, the physician should probe into whether the patient is predominantly leading a happy and peaceful life. Any negative psychological factors that lead to stress, for instance, can have a negative impact on the patient's overall health and outlook. This is especially the case when the patient becomes chronically-ill since such a patient becomes increasingly prone to experiencing even more negative emotions because (s)he is in constant pain and fatigued. Thus, through an empathic understanding of the patient's life situation, the physician can assess the chronically-ill patient's psychological states. The more the physician strives to gain an empathic understanding of the patient's unique situation, the more the physician will understand about the patient's unique situation.

Second, the decision in favour of a treatment should be made by the patient in conjunction with the physician. The chronically-ill patient should always strive to openly communicate his/her medical needs to the physician. It is essential that the physician become reflexively aware of the patient's medical concerns and any familial idiosyncrasies, such as whether there is a manipulative spouse, financial difficulties, and so on. Stress can wreak havoc with a chronically-ill patient's ability to cope with continuous pain and fatigue may even increase the patient's disability. Therefore, this kind of empathic interaction can help the physician become more aware of what the patient has to cope with on a daily basis and how to help the patient deal with it in the most effective way possible.

Third, the patient's request for treatment must be continuous, conscious, reflective and freely made. There is so much room for abuse in this area that it is essential for a physician to empathically communicate directly with the chronically-ill patient about this matter. This will ensure that the patient is making a rational decision which is informed and unbiased by relatives and family. Many times, family members or relatives may pressure patients to undergo treatments they wouldn't agree to themselves. If a patient feels pressured, (s)he should stand back for a while before making a decision. If the patient is depressed, (s)he should be prescribed antidepressants, and wait for a while before making a decision. In this way, the physician can be as responsive as possible to the patient's needs. However, if the patient makes continuous and consistent requests in favour of a particular treatment, and (s)he is rational, and the decision doesn't appear to be biased by third parties, then his/her request in favour of or against a treatment should be considered genuine.

Fourth, the physician should empathically determine whether or not the patient's pain and suffering can be relieved in other ways. Sometimes, there are other less invasive medical treatments that the patient could try first. For example, a chronically-ill patient's illness may not be progressing as quickly as initially anticipated. Therefore, the patient may not need to undergo invasive treatments, such as hip replacement surgery. The physician can simply prescribe more pain medications in the interim. However, before the physician can make such an assessment, (s)he should be empathic with the patient's pain and suffering by imagining *what it would be like* to be in the patient's predicament. In other words, the physician must ask him/herself: *How would I feel if I was in so much pain all the time? What would I do? How would I cope?* This will give the physician an idea of how desperate and perhaps frustrated the patient may be feeling.

# Conclusion

Thus, given the nature of chronic illness, many times, patients make decisions in favour or against treatment which are counterintuitive and sometimes even biased. The physician should always determine whether or not the patient should be *guided* to successfully make important decisions. This does not mean that the physician must make a decision on the patient's behalf. The physician's role is merely one of *guiding* the patient's thinking processes of the patient so that (s)he could make a rational decision that is free from biases and negative feelings. Thus, the physician should merely fulfill the role of mentor and collaborator of decision-making for patients. Some physicians still resist shared decision-making because of the time constraints involved in such a practice. However, shared decision-making can sometimes save a patient undue hardship and ensure that (s)he is making a rational decision about future interventions. So, it is time well-spent.

Thus, physicians may need to spend a substantial amount of time guiding some of their patient's thinking processes. As we saw, some chronically-ill patients may lack the kind of reflective awareness that is necessary to make the most effective assessments about treatment. The physician should not expect the patient to proceed on his/her own since, given his/her chronic condition, that patient may lack the kind of objective reflection that is necessary to make a rational decision. This requires that the physician and patient engage in shared communication in order to reach the most rational decision about a treatment. Effective communication, in turn, requires that an open, honest physician–patient relationship is developed and nurtured by the physician. I turn to this topic in the next chapter.

# Chapter 8

# Developing an Effective Physician–Patient Relationship

The fourth condition of a patient-centered approach for the chronically-ill is for the physician to take steps to develop and nurture an effective physician–patient relationship. To bring this condition about, the physician must have an awareness of the chronically-ill patient's values and life goals. Every chronically-ill patient will have different needs for information-disclosure about his/her illness, depending on his/her psychological and personal needs. Unless the physician is aware of these differences in advance, (s)he will not be able to effectively disclose the relevant information about the treatments to the patient.

Likewise, the chronically-ill patient must also become more cognizant of the physician's attitudes towards certain aspects of his/her illness. For instance, if a physician is in the habit of being impatient to talk to a patient about her continuous pain or fatigue, the physician will probably not take these symptoms seriously.

Open and honest communication is difficult to bring about if the physician doesn't disclose all the treatment options available to the patient. To develop an effective physician–patient relationship, the patient must trust that the physician has disclosed all the information about the treatments. In addition, the physician must trust that the patient has understood all the treatments and can make a rational decision about treatment. This reciprocal relationship of trust and openness is one of the building blocks for developing an effective physician–patient relationship.

In this chapter, I will argue that there are two central components of an effective physician–patient relationship: effective disclosure, and shared decision-making. Shared decision-making is impossible to achieve without honest, open, non-manipulative communication between the patient and physician. A physician who uses manipulative techniques to convince the patient to undergo a particular treatment undermines the patient's trust which can further hinder the development of an effective physician-patient relationship.

# Treatment Disclosure Without Manipulation

For humane health care to be practiced most effectively, the exchange between physician and patient must be free from manipulative techniques. Such techniques may lead patients to make forced decisions that are substantially uninformed. Rather, the treatments must be presented to the chronically-ill patient in an objective manner (i.e., free from psychological manipulations) which takes into account the patient's values and long and short-term life goals.

The three kinds of manipulations that can be used by physicians from time to time are: (1) Coercion; (2) Persuasion; and (3) Tone of voice. I will examine each of these below.

## Coercion

Coercion is defined as the intentional influences that pose or exaggerate a credible threat of unwanted and avoidable harm, so influential that the chronically-ill patient cannot resist avoiding it. In such a case, the chronically-ill patient would be consenting to treatment that is not necessarily freely chosen, and hence the decision made would be uninformed. This occurs most notably when the physician decides that the patient should undergo a particular medical treatment without taking the patient's unique values and life goals, life situation or even his/her previous medical history into consideration. If the chronically-ill patient unreflectively accepts a particular treatment, (s)he simply agrees with the physician's recommendations. This cannot be considered an informed choice in favor or against treatment.

Few physicians consciously use coercive techniques due to the irrational responses which occur for the patient. Physicians only use coercion as a last resort if they believe that the patient is refusing treatment that will benefit him/her. For instance, if a chronically-ill patient refuses to undergo an elective surgery that will help him/her live with less pain in the future, sometimes the physician may try to convince the patient by saying: *If you don't have surgery, you'll probably be in a wheelchair in time.* This tactic, although it may be helpful to get the patient to undergo the surgery, can hinder the patient from making an informed choice in the short-term. It is best for the physician to allow the patient to decide for him/herself.

Instead, the physician should *guide* the chronically-ill patient's thinking so that (s)he will make a more rational decision in favor of the surgery the second time the option is presented. Some patients habitually make decisions in favour of certain treatments and avoid others. Yet, upon a second and third discussion of the treatment options, chronically-ill patients usually realize that their previous decision was indeed irrational.

## Persuasion

Persuasion may be characterized as the successful attempt to convince a patient, through appeals to reason or emotion, to undergo a treatment or surgical procedure that the physician believes will improve his/her overall health and well-being. When a chronically-ill patient's beliefs are manipulated by the physician in this way, (s)he may be persuaded to undergo a medical treatment that may not be in accordance with his/her values and life goals. This is the most problematic of the two types of manipulation since it is sometimes difficult for a chronically-ill patient to correctly ascertain whether or not (s)he is being persuasively influenced by the physician. Sometimes, the physician may persuade the patient in such a way that (s)he is unaware of even being influenced. This can destroy the trust between patient and physician.

Chronically-ill patients may also be influenced by the way the medical treatments are presented and ordered since they may believe that the treatments presented first must be the most relevant ones for their purposes. By ordering the medical treatments without the patient's consent, the physician is manipulating the patient by presenting what (s)he believes is the most viable treatment first so that the patient will most likely remember it and go along with the treatment. Most patients typically opt for one of the first treatments presented, depending on which one (s)he remembers most clearly. One solution to this problem may be for the patient to simply ask whether or not there is any importance attached to the physician's ordering of the treatments. Another way to circumvent such tactics would be for the patient to ask that the treatments be presented in written form so that (s)he could read them him/herself first. This ensures that the chronically-ill patient will first consider the recommended treatments herself prior to the appointment and then rank them with the guidance of the physician during the appointment.

## Tone of Voice

When a physician speaks in a loud tone of voice, this may give the chronically-ill patient a feeling of uneasiness. This negative feeling can force the patient to make a haphazard and unreflective decision in favour of a treatment. This may again result in the patient accepting a treatment that (s)he did not genuinely consent to. Softer voices, on the other hand, may connote acceptance and less risk. Chronically-ill patients interpret such verbal cues in a variety of ways, depending on their state of mind at the time. However, a loud tone of voice always negatively impacts a patient and can affect his/her decision-making abilities.

There are several known reasons why physicians feel justified using such manipulative techniques. These are: (i) Time constraints; (ii) Deficiency in a patient's psychological competency; (iii) A patient's inability to understand basic medical conversations; and (iv) Personality clashes. I will examine each of these in turn below.

### *Time Constraints*

Most physicians operate within many time constraints. It seems to be in the nature of medical practice for physicians to have a lot more patients every year. However, when treating chronically-ill patients, the physician must plan to take a sufficient amount of time to be able to bring about a humane clinical encounter.

### *Deficiency in a Patient's Psychological Competency*

Every chronically-ill patient has a different level of psychological competence and emotional intelligence. Most chronically-ill patients are sufficiently competent to make their own decisions about a medical treatment. Some patients, however, may be more prone to irrational thinking, and they should be *guided* by the physician more often into making an informed decision in favour of a treatment. However, under no circumstances should the physician be manipulative or coercive towards the patient. Instead, the physician should ensure that the patient's decision in favour or against a treatment is rational and reflective.

## *A Patient's Inability to Understand Basic Medical Conversations*

Some physicians believe that most patients won't understand their explanations of treatment. This need not be the case because most medical terms have an explanation in ordinary language that can be understood by most patients. However, despite this, some patients may still not understand the information disclosed. This can be very frustrating for the physician but something that can be overcome with patience.

## *Personality Clashes*

Personality clashes between physician and patient are not uncommon occurrences either. Character clashes occur when there is personal friction between physician and patient. The reasons for such clashes are usually largely unknown. Because of this, some physicians may unconsciously treat a patient in a condescending manner. Given the current focus on partnership-based relationships in medical practice, it is no longer acceptable for the physician to be condescending in any way to the patient. If personality clashes are detected by the patient, (s)he has a right to change physicians and find one that is more compatible.

However, each of these justifications can further coerce patients into medical decisions which undermine a patient's ability to making an informed decision. Thus, on the patient-centered approach advocated in this book, these rationalizations must be avoided by the physician.

# Shared Decision-Making

To develop an effective physician–patient relationship, shared decision-making is crucially important. Shared decision-making requires that both the patient and physician have an input about a particular plan of treatment. Ideally, shared decision-making divides its labour between physician and patient. Most simply defined, the physician's role is to use his/her training, knowledge, and expertise to provide the patient with facts about the chronic illness. The patient's role, on the other hand, is to rely on his/her personal preferences and life goals to evaluate the treatments, by selecting one that is best suited to his/her unique situation. However, this ideal has many challenges. The facts/values division of labour in decision-making can be hard to bring about in medical practice. It is hard to assess a treatment on the level of facts and values alone. Each level provides its own challenges. However, ideally these two levels together provide patients with the best analysis of treatment, which is one of the most important goals of shared decision-making. On the patient-centered approach advocated throughout this book, it is necessary for physicians to try to bring about shared decision-making as often as possible in medical encounters. Patients need to be consulted about the impact of a particular treatment at every juncture.

Shared decision-making consists of: (1) acknowledging uncertainty; (2) sharing authority; and (3) developing mutual trust. Shared decision-making is difficult for some medical professionals to accept because of the underlying paternalistic tradition that has been in effect in medicine for centuries. Traditionally, medicine has been viewed by the general public as a stable and reliable profession, with few known uncertainties. When a chronically-ill patient needs medical attention, it is now common for him/her to believe that the science of medicine will help him/her by lessening his/her pain and discomfort through treatments, procedures or medications. There has been a concern by many medical professionals that shared decision-making between the patient and physician may result in a public awareness of some of the uncertainties of medicine that physicians are acutely aware of but don't want to disclose. Some physicians may feel that, if the chronically-ill patient becomes aware of these uncertainties, (s)he may feel even more vulnerable and uncertain. This isn't the case for most patients, however.

## Acknowledging Uncertainty

The unknown dimensions of chronic illness make medical practice unpredictable and uncertain at times. Some physicians would prefer to keep this uncertainty hidden from their patients since they want to uphold medical certainty at all times and the trust that patients may have in medical practice as a whole. In other words, physicians want to keep their professional image intact, even if that means keeping some valuable information concealed from the patient. However, this undermines a patient's ability to make an informed decision by making it impossible for that patient to refuse treatment even if the probabilities of being helped are rather uncertain. In addition, shared decision-making is difficult, if not impossible, to bring about unless the physician fully discloses such uncertainties to the patient. By becoming aware of the success rate of a treatment, the patient will have the necessary information to make an informed decision.

## Sharing Authority

Sharing authority in decision-making does not necessarily mean that physicians and chronically-ill patients must make a *joint decision* about a medical treatment each time. A joint decision occurs when the physician and patient agree on a treatment plan. This still takes a lot of the responsibility for making such decisions away from the patient. Instead, the physician must *guide* the chronically-ill patient into non-judgmental, nonbiased and non-prejudicial decisions in favor of treatment. When a physician *guides* a patient to make the best decision, (s)he provides all the information necessary about the treatments and answers any questions that the patient may have. However, the final decision still has to be made by the patient. This process will ensure that the patient will make an informed decision in favor of a medical treatment which is ultimately the goal of shared decision-making and the patient centered approach. However, if the physician and patient do not form a partnership-type relationship in which each person *equally* contributes to the decision-making process, an informed, rational, and reflective decision about a medical treatment will be difficult to bring about.

Shared decision-making consists of developing a mutual dependency relationship between the chronically-ill patient and physician. The physician cannot disclose the information about medical treatments without the personal knowledge provided by the chronically-ill patient, and the patient cannot make a decision in favour of a treatment without an effective disclosure of medical information that is properly understood. Thus, both the patient and physician are considered to be *authorities* in different ways since the patient knows his/her personal values and life situation while the physician has the medical knowledge and expertise to help the chronically-ill patient.

## Developing Mutual Trust

For shared decision-making to occur most effectively, the chronically-ill patient and physician must trust one another. Due to the vulnerabilities of the medical profession's uncertainties and the patient's illness, mutual trust is essential to fostering a relationship where the two parties can engage in open and honest communication. Mutual trust has two dimensions, one for the physician and one for the chronically-ill patient. The patient must trust that the physician has disclosed all the information honestly and openly to ensure that (s)he can reach a rational decision in favour of a medical treatment. The physician must, in turn, trust that the patient has understood all the information about the treatments competently and can make a rational decision about the best treatment for him/her.

When I say that the physician should trust the patient, I mean that (s)he trusts that the patient is capable of reflecting sufficiently on all the relevant aspects of the treatment. This presupposes that the patient has understood all the information relayed and (s)he has clearly communicated all his/her difficulties to the physician in order that these may be addressed in detail. This trust may take the form of an intuition on the part of the physician about the chronically-ill patient. The patient and physician must develop this type of mutual trust and respect over time for the clinical encounter to be most effective.

Building mutual trust and respect between patient and physician is an essential condition for establishing a humane physician–patient relationship. It can take a substantial amount of time, and effort for both the physician and patient to develop such a trusting relationship. The trust that is developed between the physician and patient requires more than a mere recognition that the physician has the medical expertise to perform the treatment effectively. In addition, physicians should not hesitate to share their difficulties in decision-making with their patients. This can further open up lines of communication between the patient and physician.

However, trust and respect between the chronically-ill patient and physician are not easily acquired virtues in medical practice. Physicians must strive to give both a diseased body and diseased person proper recognition and where conflicts arise, they must reconcile whether they will give preference to the diseased body or diseased person. Within the patient-centered approach presented in this book, a diseased person takes precedence over the diseased body. In other words, there is no necessary boundary between the body and the person since whatever happens to the body always influences the person in some way. Thus, the physician must ideally focus on both the physical and psychological dimensions of a patient's illness.

# Conclusion

In this chapter, I discussed the importance of developing an effective physician–patient relationship to bring about the patient-centered approach. One of the chief features of developing such a relationship is to effectively communicate and engage in shared decision-making. This presupposes the development of mutual trust and respect between physician and patient. Thus, a patient-centered approach cannot be developed without fostering an effective physician–patient relationship. In the next chapter, I will discuss the importance of advocating humane health care for a chronically-ill patient.

# Chapter 9

# A Humane Patient-Centered Approach

The purpose of this chapter is to assess the patient-centered approach for the chronically-ill patient in terms of the four conditions outlined in the previous chapters. As has been argued in the book, the patient-centered approach is especially necessary for the chronically-ill patient since many times such a patient is unable to make unbiased decisions in favour or against treatments. It is, therefore, essential that the physician bring about the four conditions of a patient-centered approach to health care outlined in this book to provide the most humane and effective patient care.

A chronically-ill patient usually has three possible options for treatment or medical intervention. In some cases, both of these options are necessary to provide the most relief to a chronically-ill patient. First, the patient can undergo surgery to alleviate some of the immediate negative effects of disability caused by the chronic illness. Secondly, the patient can take different medications to relieve pain and other symptoms. Thirdly, the patient must change his/her lifestyle to accommodate the chronic condition. The patient will have to learn new ways to live and to pace him/herself effectively. In each of these three approaches, the patient, along with a specialist and/or medical practitioner, has to decide which treatments or self-management techniques are the best to work towards. I will discuss each of these options in detail in this chapter.

To this end, this chapter will fulfill two main purposes. First, I will show how the patient-centered approach is necessary to administer humane health care for the chronically-ill. I will argue that without the patient's personal and psychological information, the physician cannot effectively prescribe the best treatments for the patient since the subjective aspect of the prognosis is missing. Second, I will show that there are two foundational components of the patient-centered approach. First, the patient and physician should feel sufficiently comfortable with each other to openly and honestly discuss the patient's medical situation in a trustworthy manner. Second, the patient and physician should develop a partnership-type relationship. Without the development of this type of relationship, a chronically-ill patient's care cannot be brought about in any kind of meaningful way. And by developing a partnership-type relationship, physicians can encourage patients to engage in several self-management practises that will help them substantially.

# The Patient-Centered Approach and the Meaning of Chronic Illness

The traditional paradigm of medicine views the patient's illness as a diseased body that can be cured by using various kinds of treatment and/ or surgery. For the physician, a diseased state is an entity that can be separated from the patient experiencing the illness. According to the patient-centered approach, although the illness is part of the patient's body, it also substantially affects the patient's quality of life. This is especially the case for chronic illness. The difference between a physician's narrative of illness as a disease and the patient's as a lived experience highlights the reason why the patient and physician cannot effectively communicate with one another. The four conditions of the patient-centered approach outlined in the book propose ways to break these barriers to effective communication between the physician and patient by including objective and subjective factors of medical care.

In order for the physician to most effectively and humanely treat the patient, the physician must shift focus from the diseased state of a patient's body to the change in quality of life experienced by the chronically-ill patient. This requires the physician to shift his/her focus from the objective features of the disease to the subjective, personal ones during the clinical encounter. When a physician interprets a chronic illness as merely a diseased state, s(he) separates the patient's diseased body from the self. However, the patient's diseased body and self are both negatively impacted by a chronic illness, and a physician cannot effectively prescribe treatments without treating both the patient's body and mind. This presupposes that the physician must pay particular attention to the physical and psychological changes that the patient is experiencing as a result of his/her illness. Physicians must, therefore, spend a considerable amount of time during the clinical encounter discussing the impact that a particular chronic illness has on the patient's quality of life. Therefore, an important part of treating a chronically ill patient is encouraging him/her to persevere and gain the courage to resume his/her normal daily activities, despite his/her physical disabilities.

Thus, the meaning of illness, as experienced by the patient, has subjective overtones. This doesn't mean that the patient cannot express the pain (s)he is experiencing in a way that can be effectively understood by the physician. A patient understands what an illness means to his/her life, when (s)he determines how it negatively impacts different aspects of his/her life. This sense of meaning presupposes a unique kind of particularity. For instance, when a chronically-ill patient experiences pain and fatigue for an extended period, the patient's narrative will be subjective in that (s)he will report the particular impact that the pain and fatigue has had on his/her body, and especially quality of life. The patient may say, *"I used to walk a half an hour a day, three times a week, and now I can only walk for fifteen minutes. And even then I have a lot of pain and I feel very tired when I get back."* This narrative assessment highlights the subjective impact of the illness on the patient's life. Recognition of the subjective aspects of a patient's illness is essential for the physician to determine the best treatments for the patient.

# The Four Conditions of the Patient-Centered Approach Revisited

As we discussed in Chapters 5 to 8, the patient-centered approach consists of developing four conditions: (1) Empathic Communication; (2) Effective Understanding; (3) Successful Decision-making; and (4) Developing a Trusting Physician–Patient Relationship. As will be seen below, there is symmetry between the components of humane medicine and the four conditions of the patient-centered approach. In other words, without the patient-centered approach, human health care cannot be fully achieved.

## Empathic Communication

In Chapter 5, I discuss condition one of a patient-centered approach which requires that a physician must clearly and empathically communicate the diagnosis, prognosis, and treatment options to the patient. This can be achieved by focusing on the patient's narrative of illness. In other words, after the diagnosis, prognosis and treatment options are disclosed, the physician must carefully and empathically listen to the chronically-ill patient's story of illness. A patient's life is usually negatively impacted by a chronic illness. Nothing is the way it used to be, including how the patient feels from day-to-day. The chronically-ill patient may feel increasingly disabled, weak, and more in pain as time goes on. Further, the treatments may not initially be beneficial but merely causing further negative side effects. All of these aspects of a chronically-ill patient's experience of illness should be carefully taken into consideration by the physician.

The physician must empathically and individually assess the prognosis of every chronically-ill patient's illness. Statistics may give the physician a better idea of the frequency of a particular chronic illness, given a patient's age group, life situation, and genetics. However, each patient's life must be treated as intrinsically unique and different, thereby posing different challenges. A patient's condition should never be evaluated merely in a statistical manner. As each patient will experience the chronic illness differently, (s)he will cope with the illness in unique ways as well. Physicians should pay attention to the psychological aspects of the chronic illness since they can impact a patient's well-being more than the physical ones.

In addition, the treatments available to the patient must be disclosed clearly and concisely by the physician. Without an open and honest disclosure of the diagnosis, prognosis, and treatment options, the patient cannot give an informed consent for or against a treatment. In addition, the physician must disclose all the risks for a particular treatment. If the physician does not know if a particular treatment will be beneficial for the particular patient, (s)he should directly disclose such uncertainties to the patient. This will help to open up the discussion quite a bit and develop trust. Further, the physician should also disclose the success rates of certain procedures based on past records. This may help the patient make a more informed choice about treatment.

## Effective Understanding

As I argued in Chapter 6, I discuss the second condition of the patient-centered approach which argues that one way of developing an effective and honest physician–patient relationship is by fostering *shared understanding*, one that is based on a reciprocal understanding between patient and physician. Ordinary understanding substantially differs from reciprocal understanding since the former merely requires that the physician communicate the available treatments to the patient whereas the latter takes the patient's personal needs and values into consideration. According to the patient-centered approach, it is insufficient for the physician to merely communicate the brute facts of the treatments without *personalizing* them to the patient's needs, values, and long and short-term life goals. The personal features of a patient's treatments must be determined by the physician through shared understanding.

The physician must become aware of how the patient is personally coping with the illness. Each chronically-ill patient will experience many different negative and positive emotions during the course of his/her chronic illness. Also, patients have different coping styles. Some patients may become angry and depressed while others will insist on coping with the pain and fatigue proactively. Thus, a physician must discuss the patient's feelings in relation to his/her chronic illness and any fears and future expectations that (s)he may have. If the physician detects that the patient is depressed, (s)he should encourage the patient to see a counsellor or perhaps prescribe anti-depressant medication.

Without shared understanding and mutual trust and respect, an open, honest physician–patient relationship becomes impossible to develop. Because of the inherent vulnerabilities of the chronically-ill patient, the physician must understand and empathize with the chronically-ill patient's predicament in order for humane medicine to be achieved. This recognition should facilitate the physician's understanding and hopefully lead to a reciprocal understanding of the patient's predicament. The physician must, therefore, always facilitate an open, honest dialogue through which a patient's fears are openly discussed and uncertainties of treatment and prognosis communicated.

Thus, the physician must strive to develop a partnership-type relationship with the patient. On the one hand, the physician cannot determine the patient's values and life goals in relation to the disease without talking to the patient at length. On the other hand, the patient needs the physician to provide the medical expertise necessary to help the patient deal with the illness. The longer a patient endures pain and fatigue, the more vulnerable will (s)he feel. Thus, the physician will need to provide both psychological and physical support to the patient.

## Successful Decision-making

In Chapter 7, I discuss the third condition of the patient centered approach is the importance of ensuring that the patient makes a successful decision for treatment in a rational and level-headed manner that is consistent with his/her values, goals, and life plans, and one which is not influenced by biases and prejudices which are irrelevant to the decision being made. It is essential, therefore, for physicians to *guide* a patient's decision-making, especially when important treatment choices (such as surgery) must be made. If a chronically-ill patient is on medication, in constant pain, or experiencing extreme fatigue, this may further negatively impact his/her ability to think clearly and rationally. In such cases, the physician should either advise the patient to stop taking the medication before making an important medical decision, or *guide* the patient to ensure that his/her ultimate decision in favor of or against treatment is rational. To '*guide*' means to '*think along with*' the chronically-ill patient, encouraging him/her to deliberate rationally and reflectively. This process is typically most effective when physicians ask the chronically-ill patient some specific questions about the treatments in order to ensure that (s)he has, in fact, fully understood them during the disclosure.

Therefore, the physician must carefully listen to each patient's narrative of illness. Every chronically-ill patient has a life story to which his/her illness belongs. It is part of the patient-centered approach to allow these narratives to properly guide medical interventions. For instance, the patient may have a stressful life living with a difficult and/or abusive spouse for a long time, or may have been a smoker and overweight. All of these conditions can negatively contribute to the patient's chronic condition. It is extremely important for the physician to assess any psychological and physical reasons for illness that may exist and to take steps to help alleviate them, if possible.

## Developing a Trusting Physician–Patient Relationship

In Chapter 8, I discuss the fourth condition of a patient-centered approach for the chronically-ill in which it is essential for the physician to take steps to develop and nurture an effective physician-patient relationship. To bring this condition about, the physician must have an awareness of the chronically-ill patient's personal idiosyncrasies. Every chronically-ill patient will have different needs for information-disclosure about his/her illness, depending on his/her psychological and personal needs and goals. Unless the physician is aware of some of these differences in advance, (s)he will be unable to effectively disclose the relevant information about the possible treatments available to the patient.

Open and honest communication is difficult to develop if the physician doesn't disclose all the treatment options available to the patient. To develop an effective physician–patient relationship, the patient must trust that the physician has disclosed all the information about the treatments openly. In addition, the physician must trust that the patient has understood all the possible treatments and can make a rational decision in favour of or against treatment on the basis of this information. As I have argued, this reciprocal relationship of trust and openness is one of the building blocks for developing an effective physician–patient relationship.

# Humane Health Care

For humane health care to be practiced, the verbal exchange between physician and patient must be free from manipulative techniques such as coercion, persuasion, tone of voice, and prioritizing the treatments without the patient's awareness or consent. Such techniques may lead to forced decisions that are substantially uninformed. Rather, the treatments must be presented to the chronically-ill patient in an objective manner (i.e., free from psychological manipulations) which takes into account the patient's values and life goals.

In addition, the physician must become aware of some of the particular qualitative features of the illness and how they will impact the patient's life. Chronic illness usually negatively affects a patient's goals, career, and hobbies. It can also strain familial relationships and substantially restrict a patient's normal activities. It is, therefore, essential for the physician to become aware of the patient's unique situation so that (s)he can best help the patient recalibrate his/her life. Immediately after the diagnosis, the patient is unable to effectively cope with the symptoms of illness. Thus, the physician should encourage the patient to keep doing the activities which (s)he loves and enjoys that for as long as possible.

This will also help the patient better accept his/her chronic condition since (s)he will learn how to fit his/her life to the medical situation and yet still keep living her best life.

# Encouraging Patients to Proactively Manage Their Condition

There are many things that physicians could do to encourage chronically-ill patients, depending on how open and receptive patients are to proactively managing their lives. Some chronically-ill patients will want to do anything they can to break the pain cycle. Other patients won't be as open to helping themselves and being proactive to lessen pain and disability.

Here are a few ways that physicians could encourage patients to become more proactive about their health and break the cycle of frustration and anxiety.

First, physicians should encourage patients not to be defined by the constant pain they experience. Instead, patients should try to pace themselves and revise how they live in order not to overdo it. For instance, a chronically-ill patient may not be able to clean the whole house at once as (s)he used to. However, the patient probably can spend ten or fifteen minutes vacuuming and then take a break. This really may be difficult for chronically-ill patients to accept at first but their overall health and well-being depends upon it. Constant overexertion can create further disabilities and increased fatigue for chronically-ill patients, adding to the frustration and inability to cope. Patients must accept the fact that their lives will never be the same as they were before the onset of their chronic illness.

Thus, the unpredictable nature of chronic pain frustrates patients. Life is an uphill battle when a patient lives in constant pain. Some patients expect the pain to get worse. This can make the patient feel hopeless and out of control. However, this is not always the case. Sometimes, pain and the disability of chronic illness can stabilize for years. Therefore, patients should not negatively frame their prognosis and expect the worse to happen. Many times these negative feelings can become self-fulfilling prophecies. In other words, if the patient believes bad things will happen, they sometimes do. This negative framing of the illness and disability can also make it difficult for the patient to effectively cope with the disease. Most of the difficulty in accepting any chronic illness hinges on coming to terms with the constant pain, increased disability and the inability to do things that were so easy to do before. This can become a never-ending negative cycle if the patient isn't careful.

Second, physicians should remind patients that the illness will not always be at its worse. There will be times that the patient will feel much less pain and will be more capable of coping with the illness. And this can help the patient do some of the things that (s)he couldn't do before the onset of the illness, given his/her current pain and fatigue levels. It is, therefore, important for patients not to give up hope and stay as positive as possible. So many times, chronically-ill patients are unable to cope with their illness, and feel even more miserable.

It is important for a patient to be able to effectively cope with a chronic illness. A chronically-ill patient can develop a positive attitude by living in the present and focusing on one day at a time. Chronically-ill patients should try to live to the fullest and not concern themselves about some of the things that they cannot control. In addition, chronically-ill patients should try to avoid having a gloomy attitude towards their disease. Even the simplest tasks will be difficult for chronically-ill patients to perform on a bad day. But not every day will be a bad day. So keeping positive is crucially important for the overall quality of life of the patient.

Third, a physician should encourage the patient to develop a consistent exercise program. There is nothing that will help a patient more if (s)he moves for 20 to 30 minutes most days. However, it has to be the correct exercise and in the right quantities for it to be most effective. Otherwise, it could make a patient's pain level worse. It is therefore essential for the patient to start any exercise regimen slowly and build activity into his/her life in small increments. Only then can the patient reap the benefits of exercise. When a chronically-ill patient exercises, (s)he releases feel-good endorphins which can help him/her feel much more capable of coping with the illness. This change in attitude from negative to positive is very important for a chronically-ill patient who is struggling to cope with a never-ending cycle of pain on a daily basis.

Fourth, a physician should recommend that the patient start physiotherapy treatments to become more flexible and mobile. Many times, physiotherapy can substantially alleviate a patient's pain and discomfort by improving his/her mobility and range of motion. Also, physiotherapists will apply heat and cold to the painful area to lessen pain and inflammation. This can help a patient feel better over time. Lastly, physiotherapists can suggest flexibility and strengthening exercises which will help patients feel more flexible and supple. Usually, the more flexible a patient feels the less pain she will experience. This can help the patient feel better overall and much more able to cope with his/her chronic condition on a daily basis.

Fifth, the physician can encourage the patient to go for a massage once a month or so to help learn how to relax and release tense muscles. A tense muscle can cause the patient a lot of pain while a relaxed one can help him/her feel much more relaxed which usually translates into less pain. Therapeutic message can also help improve a patient's circulation. Good massage therapists seem to have a healing touch. Patients need to find a therapist that they are comfortable with and who can help them feel more relaxed and calm. This may mean that the patient has to try several masseuses until (s)he finds the best one for him/her.

Sixth, the physician may suggest that the patient schedule an appointment with a counsellor if the patient has serious bouts of depression. Some chronically-ill patients become depressed because of their constant pain and disability. This can cause the patient to feel out of control and pessimistic about the future. If these negative feelings continue, the patient may start feeling quite depressed. Also, if the patient is experiencing depression, (s)he will need a lot of support. Counsellors can help the patient by suggesting coping strategies so that the patient's state of mind changes and she becomes more positive over time.

# Conclusion

The chronically-ill patient requires a different kind of attention and care than acutely ill patients. Chronically-ill patients will see the physician for years about problems that have no clear-cut resolutions or cures. Thus, physicians need to treat chronically-ill patients in a very different manner from other patients. Many times, empathy and kindness can help more in treating chronically-ill patients than prescribing medications. The goals of medicine are very different for the chronically-ill patient. Physicians have to look more to the subjective side of medical practice which primarily focuses on the patient, and how her quality of life can be improved. This kind of care cannot be measured. But it can be felt.

Ideally, the patient-centered approach will help the patient feel more cared for and the physician less frustrated. I hope this book will help all chronically-ill patients feel more in control of their illness and the physician to better treat such patients. One important theme of this book is that medical practice has to be reframed to a certain degree and stretched beyond the objective, measurable components of medical practice. However, if physicians adhere to the patient-centered approach, they should be able to treat chronically-ill patients in a humane manner, one that is meaningful and can improve their patient's quality of life. Now that is a winning combination.

The four conditions outlined throughout the book are essential to provide a humane, patient-centered approach to treating a chronic illness. Without adhering to these conditions, the patient usually cannot rationally decide on the treatments which are best for him/her. This undermines a patient's decision-making abilities and can lead to an unfulfilled life. The patient must ultimately learn how to live the best life that she can with the chronic illness. There are many things that a chronically-ill patient could do to help him/herself live a better quality of life. It is up to the patient to create this kind of life for him/herself with the help of the physician. The patient-centered approach can substantially help in this regard.

# Bibliography

Abu-Saad, Huda. *Evidence-Based Palliative Care: Across the Life Span.* Oxford: Blackwell Sciences Ltd., 2001.

Aring, Charles, D. "Sympathy and Empathy." *The Journal of the American Medical Association.* Volume 167(4), (1958), 448–452.

Barnard, David, Towers and Anna, Boston, Patricia, Lambrinidou, Yanna. *Crossing Over: Narratives of Palliative Care.* Oxford: Oxford University Press, 2000.

Beauchamp, T., & Childress, J. *Principles of Biomedical Ethics.* New York: Oxford University Press, 1979.

Bennett, Henry, L. "Trees and Heads: The Objective and the Subjective in Painful Procedures." *The Journal of Clinical Ethics,* 5(3), (1994), 149–151.

Bertakis, Klea, D., Roter, Debra, Putnam, Samuel, M. "The Relationship of Physician Medical Interview Style to Patient Satisfaction." *The Journal of Family Practice, 1991,* 32(2), 175–181.

Brody, Howard. *The Healer's Power.* New Haven and London: Yale University Press, 1987.

Brody, Howard. *Stories of Sickness.* New Haven and London: Yale University Press, 1992.

Brody, Howard "Transparency: Informed Consent in Primary Care." *Hastings Center Report.* Volume 19 (1989), 5–9.

Brown, Dan. W. "Good Decisionmaking for Incompetent Patients." *Special Supplement: Hastings Center Report.* November–December, (1994), S8–S10.

Buehler, David, A. "Informed Consent—Wishful Thinking?" *Journal of Medical and Human Bioethics.* Volume 4 (1982) 43–57.

Buller, Mary Klein, Buller David, B. "Physicians' Communication Style and Patient Satisfaction." *Journal of Health and Behavior.* Volume 28 (1987), 375–388.

Cassell, Eric. J. *The Healer's Art: A New Approach to the Doctor–Patient Relationship.* Philadelphia and New York: J.B. Lippincott Company, 1998.

Cassell, Eric. J. "The Function of Medicine." *The Hastings Center Report, (1977),* 16–19.

Coleman, Lester. L. "The Patient–Physician Relationship." *Physician's World,* 1974.

Dube, Laurette, Guylaine Ferland, D.S. Moskowitz. *Emotional & Interpersonal Dimensions of Health Services: Enriching the Art of Care with the Science of Care.* Montreal: McGill University Press, 2003.

Elias, Sherman & Annas, George J. "The Whole Truth and Nothing but the Truth?" *Hastings Center Report,* Volume 18, (1988), 35–36.

Faden, Ruth, R. & Beauchamp, Tom L. *A History and Theory of Informed Consent.* New York: Oxford University Press, 1986.

Forrow, Lachlan. "The Green Eggs and Ham Phenomena." *Special Supplement: Hastings Center Report,* November to December (1994), S29–S32.

Frankel, R.M. "Emotion and the physician–patient relationship." *Motivation and Emotion,* 1995, 19: 163–173.

Fromer, Margot, Joan. *Ethical Issues in Health Care.* St. Louis: Mosby, 1981.

Glumgart, Hermann, L. "Caring For the Patient." *The New England Journal of Medicine.* Volume 270(9), (1964), 444–456.

Greenfield, S., S.H. Kaplan, and J.E. Ware. "Expanding patient involvement in care: Effects on patient outcomes." *Annals of Internal Medicine* 102: 520–8.

Hall, Judith, A., Dornan, Michael C. "What Patients Like About Their Medical Care and How Often They are asked: A Meta-Analysis of the Satisfaction Literature." *Social Science and Medicine, 1988,* 27(9), 935–939.

Hall, J.A., T.S. Stein, D.L. Roter, and N. Rieser. "Inaccuracies in physicians' perceptions of their patients." *Medical Care* 37: 1,164–8.

Hoffman, C., D. Rice, and H.Y. Sung. "Persons with chronic conditions: Their prevalence and costs." *Journal of the American Medical Association ,* (1996) , 276: 1,473–9.

Jackson, Jennifer. "Telling the Truth." *Journal of Medical Ethics,* (1991), 17, 5–9.

Kahneman, Daniel & Tversky, Amos. "Choices, Frames and Values." *American Psychologist,* (1984), Volume 39(4), 341–350.

Kantor, Jay. E. *Medical Ethics for Physicians-in-Training.* New York: Plenum Medical Book Company, 1989.

Kaufman, M.R. "Practising good manners and compassion." *Medical Insight,* (1970), 2: 56–61.

Kohut, Nitsa, Sam, Mehran O'Rourke, Keith MacFadden, Doublas K. Salit Irving, Singer, Peter A. "A stability of treatment preferences: although most preferences do not change, most people change some of their preferences." *Journal of Clinical Ethics.* (1997), Volume 8(2), 124–135.

Levenstein, J.H. "The patient-centered general practise consultation." *South Africa Family Practice,* (1984), 5: 276–82.

Lewis, Rees, J. "Patient Views on Quality Care in General Practise: Literature Review." *Social Science and Medicine,* (1994), 39(5), 655–670.

Like, Robert, and Zyzanski, Stephen. "Patient Satisfaction with the Clinical Encounter: Social Psychological Determinants." *Social Science and Medicine,* 24(4), (1987), 351–357.

Lindemann, Nelson, Hilde, Lindemann Nelson James. "Prefrences and Other Moral Sources." *Special Supplement: Hastings Center Report.* November–December, (1994), S19–S20.

Lowenstein, Jerome. *The Midnight Meal and Other Essays about Doctors, Patients and Medicine.* Ann Arbor: The University of Michigan Press, 2005.

McCracken, E.C., M.A. Stewaret. J.B. Brown, and I.R. McWhinney. "Patient-centered care: The family practice model." *Canadian Family Physician,* (1983), 29: 2,313–16.

McCullough, Laurence and Christianson, Charles. "Ethical Dimensions of Diagnosis." *Metamedicine,* (1981), Volume 2, 129–141.

Miles, Steven, H. "Physician-Assisted Suicide and the Profession's Gyrocompass." *Hastings Center Report, 1995,* May–June, 17–19.

Minogue, Brendan, P. and Taraszewski. "The Whole Truth and Nothing But the Truth?" *Hastings Center Report, 1988,* October–November, 34–36.

Morreim, Haavi. "Three Concepts of Patient Competence." *Theoretical Medicine,* 4 (1983), 231–252.

Niemira, Denise. "Life on the Slippery Slope: A Bedside View of Treating Incompetent Elderly Patients". *Hastings Center Report,* May–June (1993), 14–17.

Novack, Dennis, H., Detering Barbara, J., Arnold Robert Forrow, Lachlan Landinsky, Morissa, and Pezullo, John, C. "Physicians Attitudes Toward Using Deception to Resolve Difficult Ethical Problems." *Journal of American Medical Association,* 261(20), (1989), 2980–2985.

Paasche-Orlow, Michael Roter Debra. "The Communication Patterns of Internal Medicine and Family Practise Physicians". *The Journal of the American Board of Family Practise,* 16 (2003), 485–493.

Payne, Sheila, Ellis-Hill, Caroline. *Chronic and Terminal Illness: New Perspectives on Caring and Careers.* Oxford: Oxford University Press, 2001.

Pearlman, Allan, Robert. "Are we asking the right questions?" *Special Supplement: Hastings Center Report.* November–December, (1994), S24–27.

Ptacek, J.T., Eberhardt, Tara, L. "Breaking Bad News: A Review of the Literature." *The Journal of the American Medical Association,* 276(6), (1996), 496–502.

Randall, Fiona, Downie, R.S. *Palliative Care Ethics: A companion for all specialities.* Oxford: Oxford University Press, 1999.

Resnik, David, B., Rehm, Marsha, Minard, Raymond, B. "The Undertreatment of Pain: Scientific, Clinical, Cultural, and Philosophical Factors). *Medicine, Health Care and Philosophy,* (2001), 4: 277–288.

Robbins, Dennis, A. *Ethical Dimensions of Clinical Medicine.* Springfield, Thomas, 1981.

Rosenberg, James, E, and Toweres, Bernard. "The Practice of Empathy as a Prerequisite for Informed Consent." *Theoretical Medicine,* 7 (1986), 181–194.

Rothenberg. R.B., and J.P. Koplan. "Chronic disease in the 1990s." *Annual Review of Public Health,* (1990), 11: 267–96.

Shelp, Earl, E. *The Clinical Encounter: The Moral Fabric of the Patient–Physician Relationship.* Dordrecht: D. Reidel Publishing Company, 1983.

Spiro, Howard, M., Curnen Mccrea, Mary G. *Empathy and the Practice of Medicine: Beyond Pills and Scapel.* New Haven: Yale University Press, 1993.

Squier, R.W. "A model of emphatic understanding and adherence to treatment regimens in practitioner–patient relationships." *Social Science and Medicine,* 1990, 30: 325–39.

Stewart, Moira. "What is a Successful Doctor–Patient Interview? A Study of Interactions and Outcomes." *Social Science and Medicine,* 19(2), (1984), 167–175.

Stewart, Moira, Brown Judith Belle, Weston, Wayne, E., McWhinney, Ian R., McWilliam Carol, L., Freeman, Thomas, R. *Patient-Centered Medicine: Transforming the Clinical Method.* London: Sage Publications, 1995.

Suchman, Anthony, L., Markakis, Kathryn, Beckman, Howard B., Frankel, Richard. "A Model of Empathic Communication in the Medical Interview." *Journal of the American Medical Association,* Volume 277(8), (1997), 678–682.

Sugarman, Jeremy. "Recognizing Good Decisionmaking for Incapacitated Patients." *Special Supplement: Hastings Center Report,* November–December, (1994), S11–S13.

Thom, David, H. and Campbell Bruce. "Patient–Physician Trust: An Exploratory Study." *The Journal of Family Practice,* (1997), 44(2), 169–176.

Tversky, Amos. "Elimination by Aspects." *Psychological Review, 1972,* Volume 79(4), 281–299.

Tversky, Amos, and Kahneman, Daniel. "The Framing of Decisions and the Psychology of Choice." *Science,* Volume 211, (1981), 453–458.

Tversky, Amos, and Kahneman, Daniel. "Judgement Under Uncertainty." *Science,* Volume 85, (1974), 1124–1131.

Veatch, Robert, M. "Abandoning Informed Consent." *Hastings Center Report,* March–April, (1995), 5–12.

Veatch, Robert, M. *A Theory of Medical Ethics.* New York: Basic Books, Inc., 1981.

Veatch, Robert, M. "Why Get Consent?" *Hospital Physician, 1975,* Volume 11, 30–31.

Wear, Stephen. *Informed Consent: Patient Autonomy and Clinician Beneficence within Health Care.* Washington, D.C.: Georgetown University Press, 1998.

Welie, Jos, V.M. Welie, Sander, P.K. "Patient Decision Making Competence: Outlines of a Conceptual Analysis." *Medicine, Health Care and Philosophy,* (2001), 4, 127–138.

White, Peter. *Biopsychosocial Medicine: An Integrated Approach to Understanding Illness.* Oxford: Oxford University Press, 2005.

Wright, Richard, A. *Human Values in Health Care: The Practice of Ethics.* New York: McGraw Hill, 1988.

# About the Author

Irene Switankowsky writes in the areas of medical ethics. She has published *A New Paradigm of Informed Consent* (1997), *A Patient-Centered Approach to Medicine for the Terminally-Ill* (2012), and *A Patient-Centered Approach to Geriatric Care* (Forthcoming) through University Press of America. She also has expertise in Philosophical Psychology and writes books for adolescents. Her most recent books are *Seasons of Empowerment for Adolescent Girls*, *The Seven Habits of Emotionally Intelligent Teens*, and *From Scattered to Unscattered Mind: A Twenty-First Century Problem*.